ELEMENTRY INTERNAL COMBUSTION ENGINE

BY

AFOFU OLUWAFEMI SULAIMON
HND (MECH IB POLY 2014) MIANG, MIRED.MNIME

PREFACE

This book is intended for student of engineering degree and diploma courses and scope in sufficiently wide range, to cover the variation in syllabus and standards of various universities and polytechnics and technical colleges. It will effectively serve as hand book, supplementing text of library reference.

AFOFU O. SULAIMON

DEDICATION

This book is dedicated to Almighty Allah, and also to the technological advancement of mankind.

ABRRREVATIONS

Generally in this hand book abbreviations will be used frequently, student will find this list useful for quick reference.

- ICE   internal combustion engine
- SIE   spark ignition engine
- CIE   compression ignition engine
- TDC   top dead center
- BDC   bottom dead center
- SAE   society of automobile engineers
- BORE   diameter of engine cylinder
- IO   Inlet valve open
- IC   Inlet valve close
- EO   Exhaust valve open
- EC   Exhaust valve close

TABLE OF CONTENT

1.0   INTRODUCTION

Automobile engine converts energy contained in fuel into relatively efficient and inexpensive transportation. Most of the modern automobile is design with internal combustion engine which are used in cars, trucks, and buses. The name internal combustion (I.C) engine is mainly classified into two which include the spark ignition engine (SIE) and the compression ignition engine (CIE). The SIE works with the mixture of air and fuel which is ignited by a spark plug and CIE works with compressed fuel at high temperature. The I.C engine is divided into two and four stroke engines. In four stroke engines the piston accomplishes four distinct strokes for every two revolution of the crankshaft. In two strokes engine there are two distinct stoke in one revolution. Variation of this engine types are used in today's automobile and include differences in number of cylinders, size and cylinder arrangement.

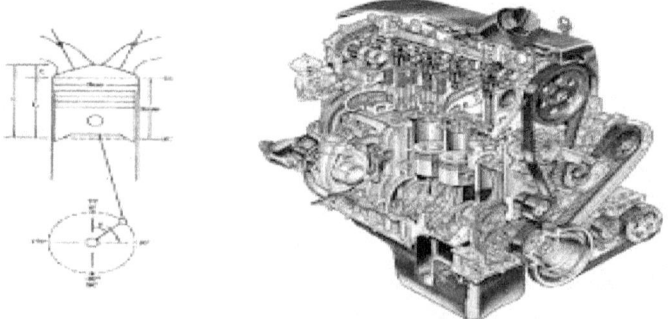

Figure 1.0 Internal combustion engine

1.1 THE EVENT ABOVE THE PISTON

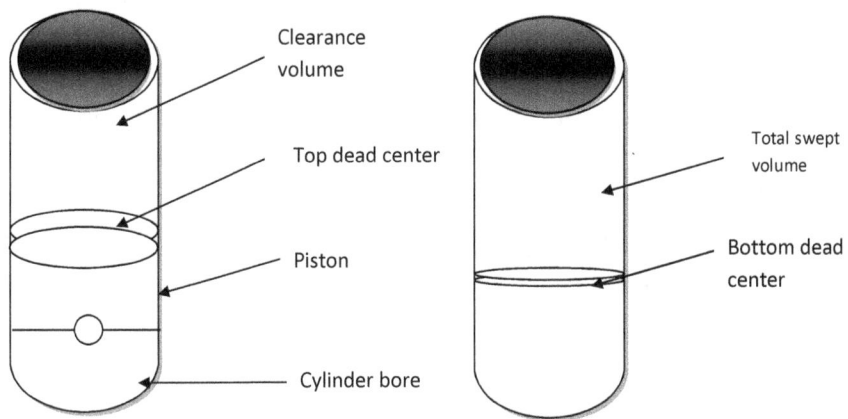

Figure 1.1 Events above the piston

1.2 ENGINE CONSTRUCTION

IC engine consist of a few large components and many small ones, most engines have more than one cylinder, It depends on the capacity of the engine produced by the manufacture. These are the major components that form up an engine.

1. Cylinder block
2. Cylinder head
3. Crankshaft
4. Piston
5. Connecting rod
6. Fly wheel
7. Cam shaft
8. Bottom tray/sump

1.2.1 CYLINDER BLOCK

This is a major component which the engine is built upon and the bore is built within were the piston is been housed. The cylinder block is mostly constructed with cast iron and aluminum alloy and variation depend on the manufacturer. The cylinder block must be rigid to hold the bore relatively to each other and hold the crankshaft in place. The crankshaft runs at right angle to the bore and being retained in the main bearing. The block form one semi circular half of the bearing and semi circular cap from the other half. The cylinder block has the engine mountain attached to outside of the motor vehicle.

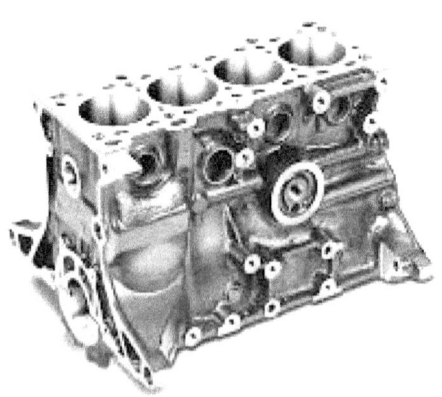

Figure 1.1 Cylinder block

1.2.2 CYLINDER HEAD

The cylinder head as the name implies it's on top of the cylinder block and it cover the cylinder block to for a combustion chamber with the machined top of the piston. The cylinder is shaped so that the combustion chamber is actually in the cylinder head. The cylinder head houses the valve, valve spring and the rocker arm, this part of the valve works via a push rods.

Sometimes the camshaft is fitted directly into the cylinder head and operates on the valve without rocker arm. This arrangement is called an overhead camshaft arrangement. The cylinder head can also be manufactured with cast iron or aluminum alloy due to the high temperature that occurs within the region. The cylinder head is been held to the cylinder block with high tensile steel stud. The joint between the cylinder block and the cylinder head must be air gas tight so that there will be complete combustion. This is achieved by using a cylinder to gasket in between the cylinder block and cylinder head.

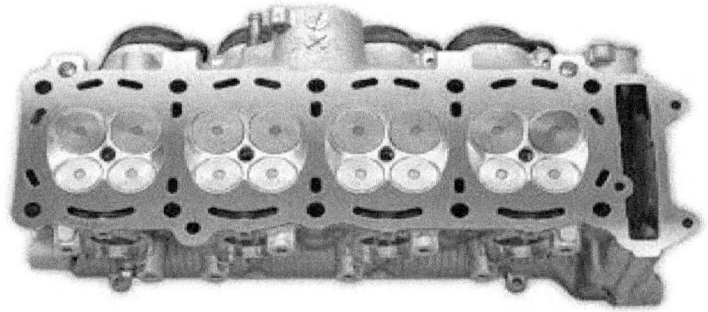

Figure 1.2 cylinder head

1.2.3 CRANKSHAFT

the crankshaft plays an important role in IC engine it work in conjuction with the connecting rod, converts the reciprocating motion of the piston to the rotary motion needed produce a certain capacity by the engine. It made from carbon steel which is alloyed with a small propotion of nickel. The main bearing jounals is fitted into the cylinder block and the big end jounals align with the connecting rods. The rear end of the crankshaft is attached to the flywheel and at the front end are the driving wheel for the timing gears, water pumps, and the cooling fan.

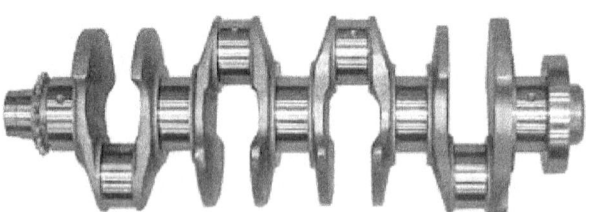

Figure 1.3 Crankshaft

1.2.4 PISTON

The piston reciprocates in the cylinder bore going form top dead center (TDC) to bottom dead center (BDC). Its purpose it to keep gases in the cylinder bore tightly sealed in place and to transmit the pressure produced when gases are burnt during the power stroke to the gudgeon pin. Piston are made from aluminum alloy, which is light, strong and good conductor of heat. They run at a speed up to 13m/s with a temperature range being as high as 2000^0c at the crown and as low as freezing point where the gudgeon pin fits. Piston sizes vary due to the capacity and the size of the engine and also work to complete the gas tighten with **the ring**.

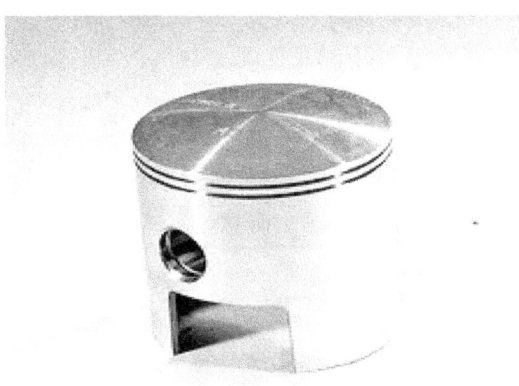

Figure 1.4 piston

The piston is mainly classified into four types.

1. PLAIN, SOLID, OPEN-ENDED

This types of very strong but heavier and has its skirt connected to it head region all the way round. It is necessary to allow clearance especially at the top of the skirt to avoid seizure.

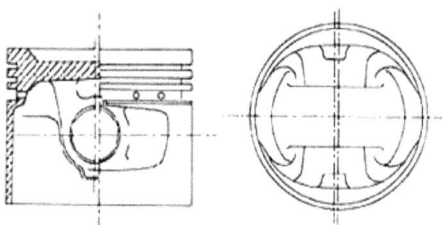

Figure 1.5 plain, solid, open-ended

2. TRANVERSE SLOT,OPEN- ENDED

Such a piston is thermally compensating and can use usually be operated at smaller clearance at the top of the skirt in the interest of noise reduction.

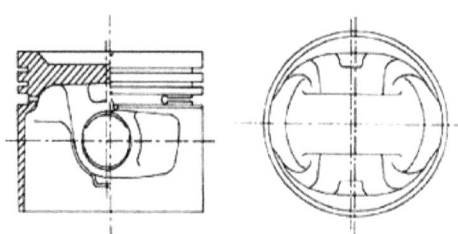

Figure 1.6 transverse slots, open ended

3. **SOLID SKIRT SLIPPER**

This type of piston has no thermal slot but the skirt is heavily cut away in the pin axis to reduce weight and avoid swaying, it is also rigid and usually needs greater clearance than other types, but this type is the strongest.

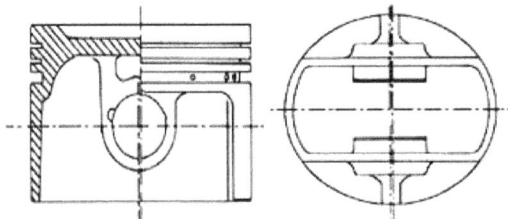

Figure 1.7 solid skirt slipper

4. **TRANVERSE SLOT SLIPPER**

Contrary to the solid skirt slipper type, this has a cast of milled transverses slot in the oil ring grove for thermal compensation. Smaller clearance at the top of the skirt is required, in the interest of less noise.

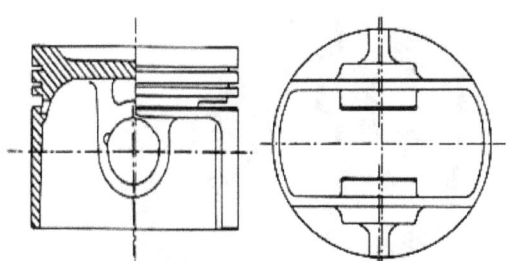

Figure 1.8 Tranverse slot slipper

1.2.5 CONNECTING ROD

The major function of the connecting rod is to connect the piston to the crankshaft, together with the crankshaft they form a simple mecanism that converts reciprocating motion into rotation motion, the might also convert in opposite side it help the piston to achive the up and down stroke in the bore. It is usually made with cast iron , a bush made from a soft metal, such as bronze is use for this joint. The smaller part go to the piston and the other end to the crankshaft.

1.7 FLYWHEEL

Flywheel is a large- diameter, heavy disk, usually constructed with cast iron. It is bolted to the engine crankshaft. The flywheel smoothies out, damps, engine vibration caused by firing pluses. It also acts as a friction surface and heat sink for one side of the clutch disk. The teeth around the circumference of the flywheel form a ring gear, which when engaged to the starter motor pinion gear are used to start the engine.

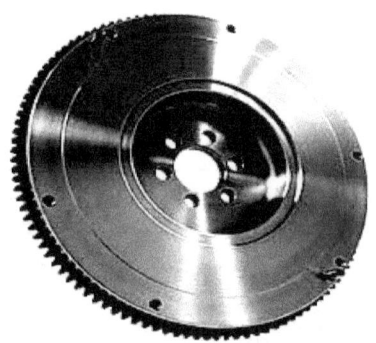

Figure 1.9 fly wheel

1.2.6 VALVE TIMING

The crankshaft and the camshaft rotations also operates the valve of the engine , the opening and closing of the valves both the inlet and the exhaust are well timed on the cam shaft rotations. the valve mechanism operates on the rotation of the camshaft lobes that open and closes the valve. The engine will and efficient performance when the appropriate mass of air and fuel enters into the combustion chamber and burn effectively. The opening and the closing of the piston in relation to the piston and crankshaft position is called valve timing.

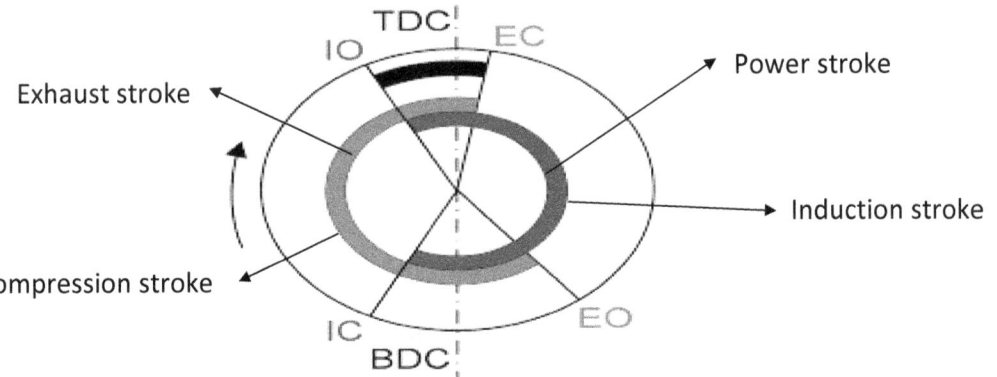

Figure 1.9.1 valve timing

1.2.7 ENGINE FIRING ORDER

The order at which the spark occurs in each cylinder is called the firing order. In order to obtain the best balance, the four the cylinder in-line engine employed crankshaft arrangement where the front and rear piston are in TDC and BDC while the center pistons are in BDC as shown below.

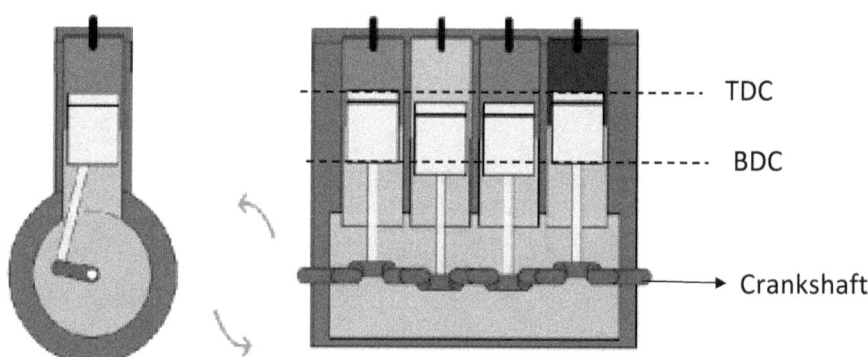

Figure 1.9.2 piston arrangement for a four cylinder engine

1st cylinder	2nd cylinder	3rd cylinder	4th cylinder	Firing order
Power	Exhaust	Compression	Induction	1
Exhaust	Induction	Power	Compression	3
Induction	Compression	Exhaust	Power	4
compression	power	induction	exhaust	2

In a four cylinder engine the firing interval will be $720^0 - \dfrac{180^0}{4}$.

The crankshaft turns twice for a complete revolution of the camshaft which is $360^0 \times 2$ that of four cylinder engine

CHAPTER 2
Types of engine cycle

2.1 Otto Cycle (SIE)

The Otto cycle is a model of the real cycle that assumes heat addition at the top of dead center. The Otto cycle consist of four reversible cycles, which is graphically shown in figure 2.0 while the four working stroke consist of the following.

1. Induction
2. Compression
3. Power
4. Exhaust

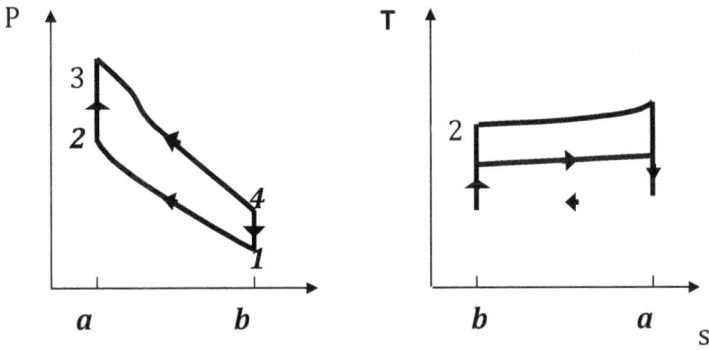

Figure 2.0 Otto cycle (p-v and t-s)

Induction stroke

The piston starts moving downward from TDC, the inlet valve opens, the displacing piston causes a partial vacuum for the intake of fresh charges (air +fuel mixture) through the inlet port into the combustion chamber, during this stroke the exhaust valve remain close.

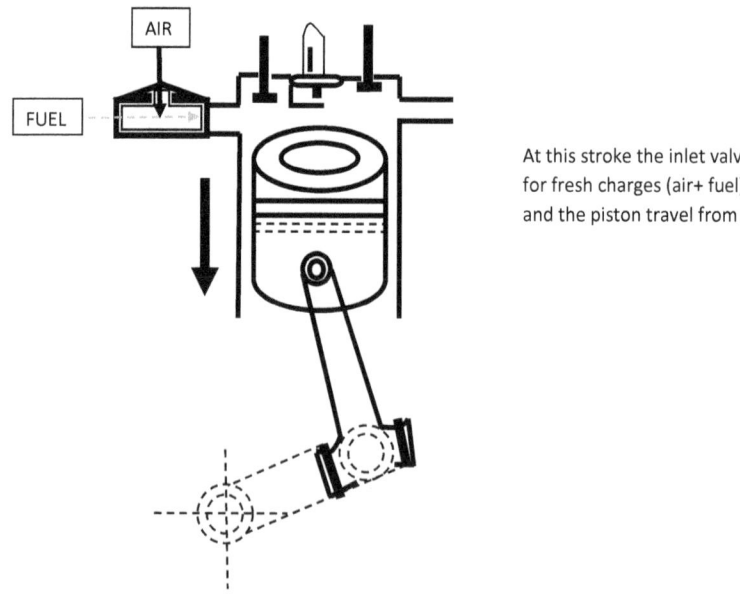

At this stroke the inlet valve will open for fresh charges (air+ fuel) to come in and the piston travel from TDC to BDC.

Figure 2.1 induction stroke

Compression stroke

At the bottom dead center (BDC) the inlet valve will close sealing the cylinder and the piston rise to compress the mixture and both valves remain close, during this stroke.

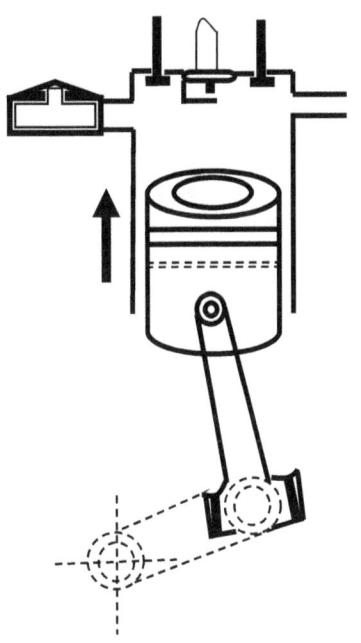

At this stroke the piston travel from BDC to TDC to compress the charges and the inlet and exhaust vale remain close.

Figure 2.2 compression stroke

Power stroke

At this stroke when the piston is close to TDC, while both valves still remain close, the compressed gas is ignited by a spark from the spark plug which will ignite the compressed gas which cause change in temperature and pressure which force the piston down to BDC.

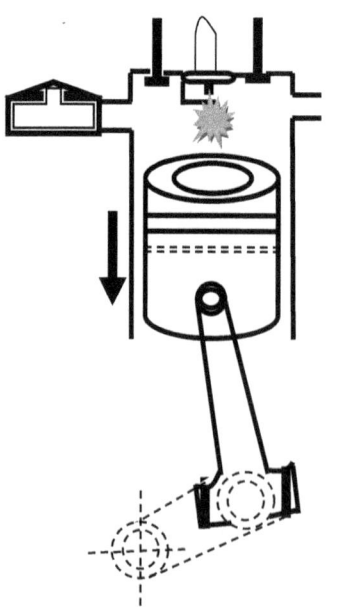

At this stroke both inlet and exhaust valves remain close the spark plug ignites a spark that forces the piston to move from TDC to BDC.

Figure 2.3 power stroke

Exhaust stroke

At bottom dead center BDC the exhaust valve open and the inlet valve closes, as the piston rises and expel out the un- burnt gas through the exhaust valve until TDC the valve closes and the piston once again commences a new induction stroke. The engine being carried over its idle strokes by the energy stored in the flywheel.

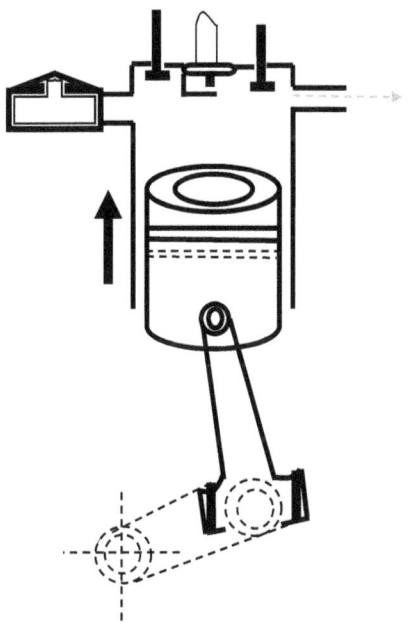

At this stroke the piston will move from BDC to TDC while the inlet vale is close and exhaust valve open to allow the un-burnt gases to go out of the combustion chamber.

Figure 2.4 exhaust stroke

2.2 Diesel Cycle

The diesel cycle is similar to Otto cycle, except that the heat addition and rejection occur at different conditions. The diesel cycle is also an ideal cycle that is it does not give an exact representation of actual process. The diesel cycle consists of four internal reversible processes. Process 1-2 is an isentropic compression. Process 2-3 is a constant pressure heat addition. This process makes the first part of the power stroke. Process 3-4 is an isentropic expansion, which makes up the rest of the power stroke. Process 4-1 finishes the cycle with a constant volume heat rejection with piston at BDC. Figure 2.5 shows the p-v and t-s diagram for the diesel cycle.

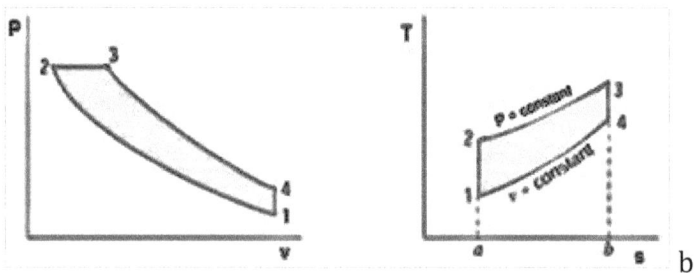

Figure 2.5 PV and TS diagram for diesel cycle

2.3 Difference between Otto and Diesel cycle

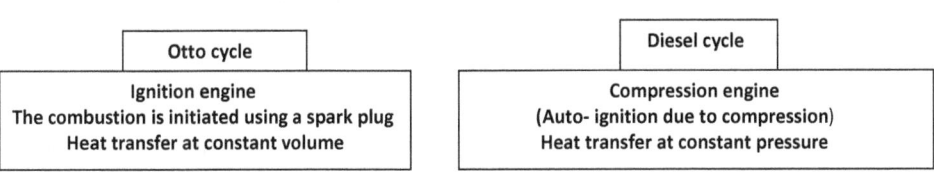

Otto cycle	Diesel cycle
Ignition engine The combustion is initiated using a spark plug Heat transfer at constant volume	Compression engine (Auto- ignition due to compression) Heat transfer at constant pressure

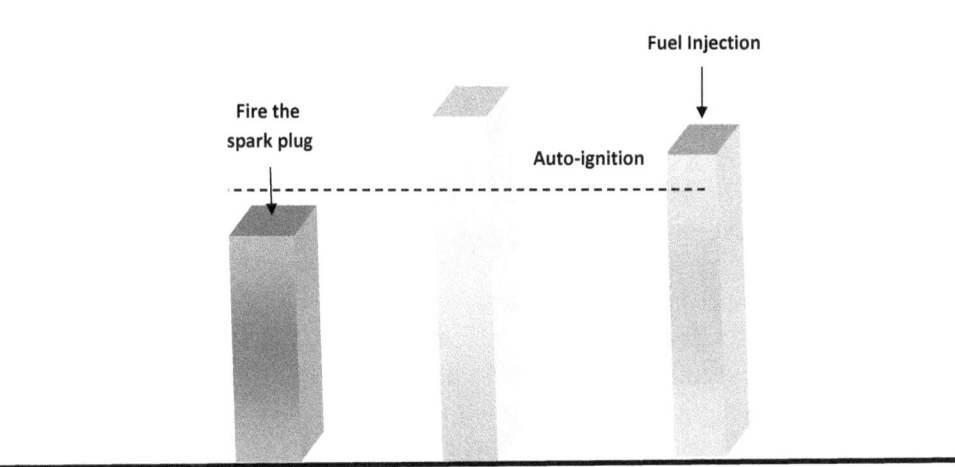

Figure 2.6 different between Otto and diesel cycle

2.4 Two Stroke Engine

The fundamental difference between the four stroke engine and the two stroke engine is the way in which the induction and exhaust process takes place.

In the four stroke engine there are separate strokes for the induction and exhaust processes. In the two stroke engine however, both the induction and exhaust processes take place with the same stroke.

The process that involves both induction and exhaust is called scavenging, or simply a gas exchange process.

The two stroke engine can be either made into a spark ignition or compression ignition engine.

The smallest engines used in two stroke engines are compression ignition engines. The engines are usually used in models and their power output does not exceed 100 W. The other type of two stroke engine with power output of up to 100 kW is spark ignition engine. Some of these engines output high power relative to their weight and bulk. Some applications of these engines are in motorcycles, chain saws and small generators.

A two stroke engine is seen in Figure 2.7. Some of the important parts of this engine are the exhaust, inlet, and crankcase port, and spark plug. The deflector is also an important design of the engine. The inlet port is where the charge is drawn from. The charge is a mixture of mainly air and fuel but may contain some exhaust. The exhaust port is where the exhaust leaves the piston, and the crankcase port provides the mixture. The combustion process for the two stroke engine goes through various processes. Following are the steps for combustion:

1) At 60^0 before hitting BDC the piston uncovers the exhaust port (EO), and the exhaust leaves the cylinder chamber while attaining atmospheric pressure. This is the end of the power stroke.

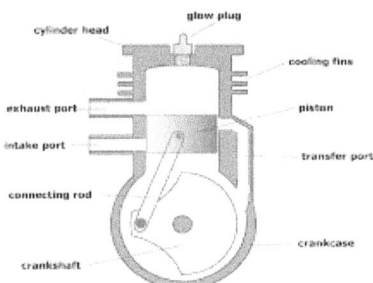

cylinder head
glow plug
cooling fins
exhaust port
piston
intake port
transfer port
connecting rod
crankcase
crankshaft

Figure 2.7 Two stroke engine.

2) At 5-10^0 later the inlet port (IO) will open and the charge that was compressed by the crankcase will flow into the main chamber and mix with some exhaust residual. Some charge will leave the exhaust port. The deflector will aid in a way that it will divert the cross flow of charge from the inlet port into the exhaust port.

3) At about 55^0 after BDC, with the piston moving up, the inlet port will now close (IC). There will be some back flow of charge from the inlet port into the crankcase.

4) At 60^0 after BDC the exhaust port will close (EC) and the piston will now compress the charge through its upward movement.

5) At 60^0 before TDC the crankcase port will open (CO) and allow charge to flow into the crankcase. The charge will flow into the crankcase since the pressure in the crankcase is below the ambient pressure.

6) When the piston is within 10-40^0 beforeTDC the charge will be compressed enough to be at a high temperature. Then combustion will follow with flame initiation from the spark plug. In this process work is done by the engine on the air and fuel mixture. The power stroke starts when the piston hits TDC and continuous until the exhaust port opens in step.

3.1 LUBRICATION

Lubrication plays a vital role in an engine system and it also promotes the performance of engine parts. The lubricating system and the cooling system help the engine to maintain a stable operating temperature. When there is contact between two surfaces friction develops because of the relative movement between the two surfaces. Friction between metals surface causes wears. To decrease friction. The two mating surface have to be separated by a lubricant. A lubricant is a thin fluid film that separates to surface so as to reduce the friction between them.

3.2 PURPOSE OF LUBRICATION

- Reduce the frictional resistance of the engine to a minimum to ensure maximum mechanical efficiency.
- Protect the engine against wear.
- Serve as a cooling agent picking up heat.
- Remove all impurities from the lubricated region.
- Form a seal between piston rings and the cylinder walls to prevent blowby.

3.3 LUBRICATION SYSTEMS

- Mist lubrication system ⎫ Two Stroke Engines.
- Wet sump lubrication system ⎤ Four Stroke
- Dry sump lubrication system ⎦ Engines

Mist lubrication system is mainly employed in two- stroke cycle engines, whereas wet and sump systems are used in four stroke cycles engine. The wet sump system is employed in relative small engines, such as automobile engines, while the dry sump system is used in large stationary, marine and aircraft engines.

3.3.1 MIST LUBRICATION SYSTEM

in two-stroke engines, the charge is compressed in the crankcase, and as such it is not suitable to have lubricating oil in the sump, therefore such engines are lubricating by adding 3% to 6% oil in the fuel tank itself. The Oil and fuel mixture is inducted through the carburetor the fuel gets vaporized and the oil in the form of mist goes into that impinges the crankcase walls lubricates the main and connecting rod bearings and the rest of the oil lubricates the piston rings and cylinder the main advantage with this system lies in the simplicity and low cost as the system does not require any oil pump filter etc.

3.3.2 WET SUMP LUBRICATION SYSTEM

In the wet sump system the bottom of the crankcase contains an oil sump (or pan) that serves as the oil supply reservoir. Oil dripping from the cylinders and bearings flows by gravity back into the wet sump where it is picked up by a pump and re-circulated through the engine lubricating system. The types of wet sump systems used are.

- The splash and circulating pump system
- The splash and pressure system
- The full force-feed system.

3.3.3 DRY SUMP LUBRICATING SYSTEM

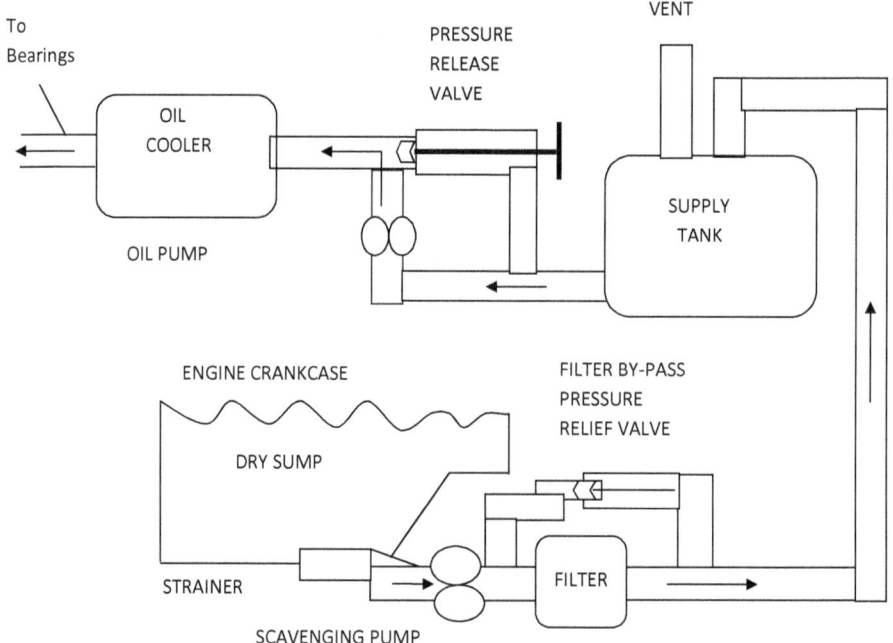

Figure 3.2 dry sump lubrication system

Dry sump lubrication system is the ultimate oiling system for internal combustion engines. The simple fact that all Formula One, Indy cars, Le Mans and Sports Racing cars as well as Super Speedway Stock Cars use dry sumps, proves this point.

The main purpose of the dry sump system is to contain all the stored oil in a separate tank, or reservoir. This reservoir is usually tall and round or narrow and specially designed with internal baffles, and an oil outlet (supply) at the very bottom for uninhibited oil supply.

3.4 PROPERTIES OF LUBRICATING OIL

- The oil used in an engine must serve as a lubricant, a coolant and an agent for removing impurities.
- It must be able to withstand high temperatures without breaking down. The oil must operate over a good range of temperature.
- The must not oxidize on the chamber walls, piston crown or at the piston rings oil should have high film strength to prevent metal-metal contact even under extreme loads.

3.5 RATING OF LUBRICATING OIL

- Lubrication oil is generally rated using a viscosity scale established by SAE.
  Commonly used viscosity grades are:
  1. SAE 5w
  2. SAE 10
  3. SAE 20
  4. SAE 30
  5. SAE 40
  6. SAE 45,
  7. SAE 50
- The oil with lower viscosity is less viscous and used in cold-weather operation. Modem high temperature high speed, close tolerance engines use high viscosity grade oil.

3.6 OIL PUMP AND TYPES

The pump's job is to draw oil from the sump and supply it with force to the moving parts of the engine. The pump must be able to force the oil into the bearing under a high pressure to keep the metal surface apart. There are three types of oil pumps commonly used in internal combustion engines.

- Gear pump
- Rotor pump
- Sliding vane pump

3.6.1 GEAR PUMP

Two gears is meshed with each other and enclosed in a aluminum pump casing. One of the gears is driven by the engine crankshaft and in turn drives the other gear.

As the gear rotate the teeth on the inlet side of the pump draw in the oil and it flows into the space left. The oil is then carried between the teeth around outer walls of the pumping chamber. When the teeth links together *again* at the outlet side of the pump the oil is squeezed out.

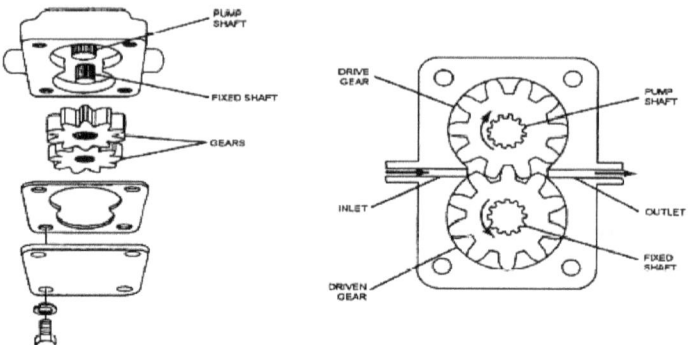

Figure 3.3   gear pump

3.6.2 ROTOR PUMP

Inside the pump there are two rotors, one inside the other. The inner rotor is mounted off-center and has one fewer lobes than the outer rotor.

The inner rotor is turned by the engine's camshaft. This turns the outer rotor at a different speed. The small space between the rotors gets larger and draws oil in through the inlet port and the large space get smaller and pump oil out through the outlet port.

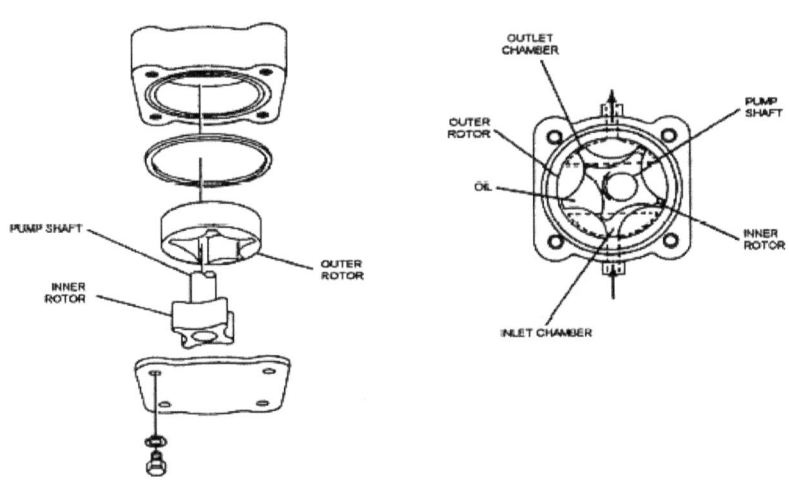

Figure 3.4 rotor oil pumps

3.6.3 SLIDING VANE PUMP

In this type of oil pimp a circular rotor is fitted off-center the pump casing. This gives a large clearance on one side, narrowing to a very small clearance on the other side. Four metal vanes are fitted in slots cuts across the surface of the rotor. These are kept in contact with the pump casing by a metal ring fitted between their inner ends.

The vane divide the chamber into four smaller chambers, which varies in size as the rotor turns, which produce the oil pumping action which is similar to the rotor oil pump.

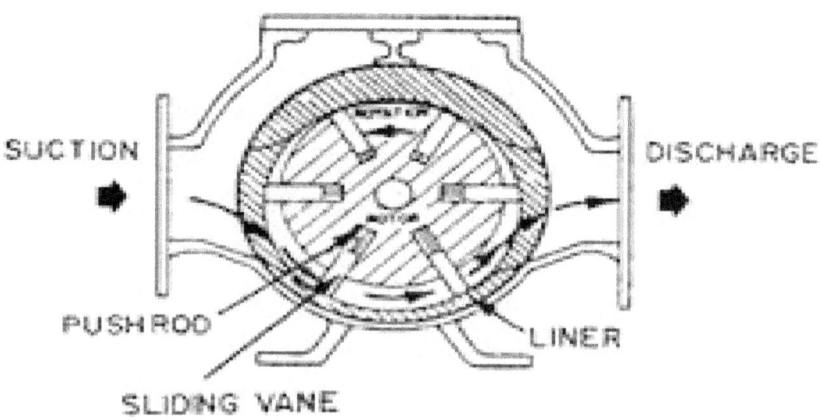

Figure 3.5 Sliding vane oil pump

4.1 COOLING SYSTEM

In internal combustion engines there are a lot of improvement in the method at which the engine is been cooled.

The major work of the cooling system it to take care of heat and also dissipate enough heat while the engine is running. It also helps to keep the engine from overheating by transferring this heat to air by a cooling fan. The car engine runs best at fairly high temperature. When the engine is cold components wear out faster and will be less efficient and emit more pollution.

There are two major type of cooling system which is named below.

- Water cooling system
- Air cooling system

4.1.1 WATER COOLING SYSTEM

The cooling system on water cooled engines circulates a fluid through pipes and passages in the engine. As the water flow through the hot parts in the engine it absorbs heat, cooling the engine. After the fluid leaves the engine it passes through a heat exchanger or radiator which transfers the heat from the fluid to the air blowing through the exchanger. In this method, cooling water jackets are provided around the cylinder, cylinder head, valve seats etc. The water when circulated through the jackets, it absorbs heat of combustion. This hot water will then be cooling in the radiator partially by a fan and partially by the flow developed by the forward motion of the vehicle. The cooled water is again recirculated through the water jackets.

4.1.2 TYPES OF WATER COOLING SYSTEM

There are two types of water cooling system which include

1. Thermo siphon system
2. Pump circulation system

Thermo siphon system

In this system water is circulated due to difference in temperature (i.e. difference in densities) of water. In this system water pump is not required but water circulates because of difference in density only.

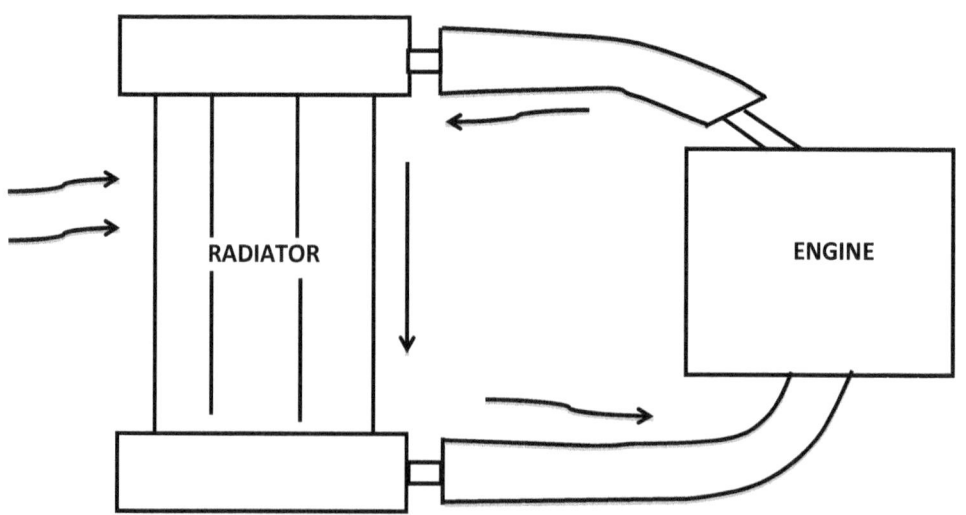

Figure 4.1 thermo siphon system of cooling

Pump Circulation System

In this system circulation of water is obtained by a pump. This pump is driven by means of engine output shaft through V-belts.

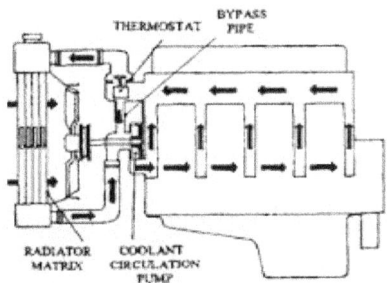

Figure 4.2 pump circulation system and component

Components of Water Cooling System

Water cooling system mainly consists of:

1. Radiator,
2. Thermostat valve,
3. Water pump,
4. Fan,
5. Water Jackets, and
6. Antifreeze mixtures.

Radiator

It mainly consists of an upper tank and lower tank and between them is a core. The upper tank is connected to the water outlets from the engines jackets by a hosepipe and the lover tank is connect to the jacket inlet through water pump by means of hose pipes.

There are 2-types of cores:

(a) Tubular core

(b) Cellular core

When the water is flowing down through the radiator core, it is cooled partially by the fan which blows air and partially by the air flow developed by the forward motion of the vehicle. As shown through water passages and air passages, water and air will be flowing for cooling purpose. It is to be noted that radiators are generally made out of copper and brass and their joints are made by soldering.

Thermostat Valve
It is a valve which prevents flow of water from the engine to radiator, so that engine readily reaches to its maximum efficient operating temperature. After attaining maximum efficient operating temperature, it automatically begins functioning. Generally, it prevents the water below 70°C.

Water Pump
It is used to pump the circulating water. Impeller type pump will be mounted at the front end. Pump consists of an impeller mounted on a shaft and enclosed in the pump casing. The pump casing has inlet and outlet openings. The pump is driven by means of engine output shaft only through belts. When it is driven water will be pumped.

Fan
It is driven by the engine output shaft through same belt that drives the pump. It is provided behind the radiator and it blows air over the radiator for cooling purpose.

Water Jackets
Cooling water jackets are provided around the cylinder, cylinder head, valve seats and any hot parts which are to be cooled. Heat

generated in the engine cylinder, conducted through the cylinder walls to the jackets. The water flowing through the jackets absorbs this heat and gets hot. This hot water will then be cooled in the radiator.

Antifreeze Mixture
In western countries if the water used in the radiator freezes because of cold climates, then ice formed has more volume and produces cracks in the cylinder blocks, pipes, and radiator. So, to prevent freezing antifreeze mixtures or solutions are added in the cooling water.

The ideal antifreeze solutions should have the following properties:
1. It should dissolve in water easily.
2. It should not evaporate.
3. It should not deposit any foreign matter in cooling system.
4. It should not have any harmful effect on any part of cooling system.
5. It should be cheap and easily available.
6. It should not corrode the system.

Advantages and Disadvantages of Water Cooling System
Advantages
1. Uniform cooling of cylinder, cylinder head and valves.
2. Specific fuel consumption of engine improves by using water cooling system.
3. If we employ water cooling system, then engine need not be provided at the front end of moving vehicle.
4. Engine is less noisy as compared with air cooled engines, as it has water for damping noise.

Disadvantages
1. It depends upon the supply of water.

2. The water pump which circulates water absorbs considerable power.
3. If the water cooling system fails then it will result in severe damage of engine.
4. The water cooling system is costlier as it has more number of parts. Also it requires more maintenance and care for its parts.

4.2 AIR COOLING SYSTEM

Air cooed system is generally used in small engines say up to 15-20 kW in internal combustion engine. In this system fins or extended surface are provided on the cylinder walls, cylinder head etc. heat is generated due to combustion processes and heat will be conducted by the fins and when air flows over the fins heat will be dissipated to the air.

The amount of air dissipated to air depends on the following
1. Amount of air flowing through the fin
2. Fins surface area
3. Thermal conductivity of the metal used for the fins

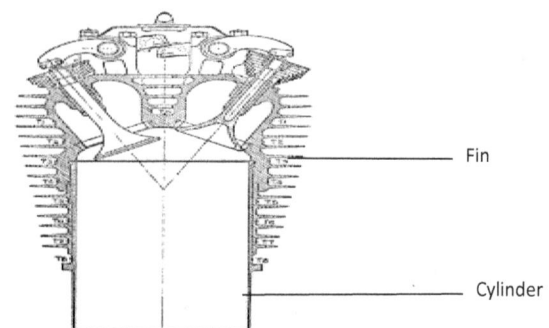

Figure 4.3 cylinder and fins

Advantages of Air Cooled System

1. Radiator and water pump is absent hence the system is light
2. Coolant and anti-freeze solutions are not requested
3. The system is the most suitable in cold climate, where if its water it may freeze.
4. In case of water there are leakages, but in this case there are no leakage

Disadvantages of Air Cooled System

1. Comparatively it is less efficient.
2. It is used in aero planes and motorcycle engines where the engines are exposed to air directly.

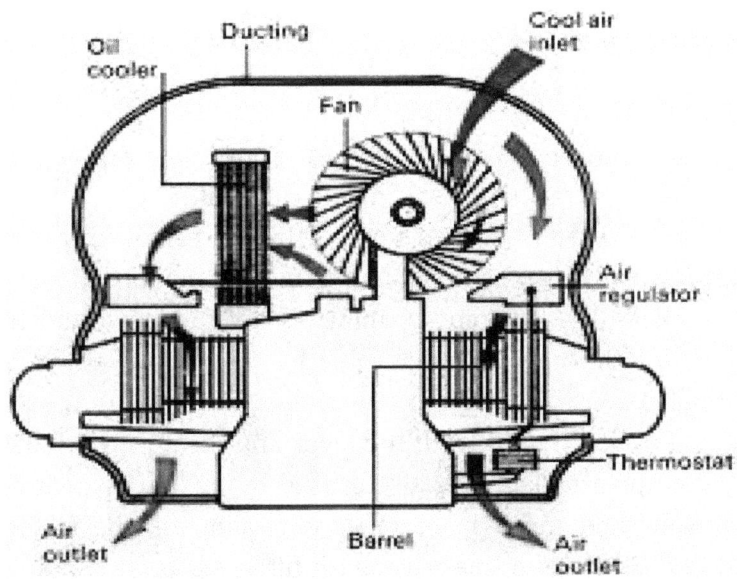

Figure 4.4 Air cooled working cycle

5.1 **FUELS SYSTEM**

In internal combustion engine the fuel (petrol and diesel) are usually stored in the tank and it convey by a pump when needed by the engine.

The tank is normally fixed far away from the engine due to the heat generated by the engine to reduce fire risk. The fuel pump helps to convey the fuel from the tank and deliver it to the unit where it will be converted to work.

It is usually fitted with a filter to stop dirt from the tank entering the carburetor or injector.

5.2 **FUEL PUMP**

There are two major types of fuel pump used in internal combustion engine.

- Mechanical pump

- Electrical pump

5.2.1 MECHANICAL FUEL PUMP

This type of pump is normally fitted to the side of the engine and it is operated by an extra cam via the engine camshaft.

The operating lever is pushed upward by the revolving cam. This through its pivot causes the diaphragm to be pulled down. The pressure inside the pumping chamber is now reduced and fuel is forced into it through the inlet valve by the normal air pressure inside the tank.

The cam revolves always from the lever and the spring pushes the diaphragm upward. The pressure caused by this movement closes the inlet valve and opens the outlet valve to allow the fuel to the unit needed in the engine. A fine wire mesh filter is usually fitted across the inlet pipe of the pump to stop dirt from the fuel tank to reach the rest of the fuel system where it could cause blockage.

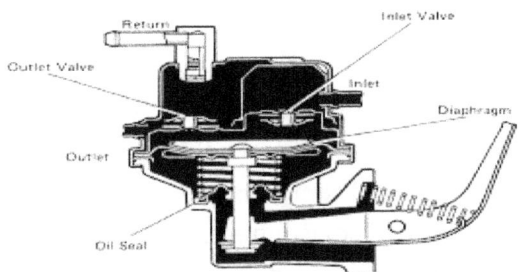

Figure 5.1 mechanical fuel pump

5.2.2 MECHANICAL PUMPS FAULTS AND THEIR CAUSES

FAULT	POSSIBLE CAUSES
Loss of pressure resulting to insufficient fuel being delivered, which may cause misfiring and loss of power at some part of the speed range and may limit engine performance.	**1.** Damage diaphragm **2.** Weak diaphragm spring **3.** Leaking valves **4.** Vapour in fuel line **5.** Broken or worn mechanical linkage
Pressure too high, causing flooding at the carburattor, increased fuel consumption and possibly stalling.	**1.** Diaphragm not properly fixed **2.** Wrong diaphragm spring

5.2.3 ELECTRICAL FUEL PUMP

The electrical fuel pump works in the same way as thed mechanical pump execp the fact that the diphargm is moved by a solenoied instead of a cam in the engine.

When electric is swiched on, the solinoied behaves like a magnet and the amature is pilled towards it.this pull the diaphagm back and fuel is drawn into the pump through the inlet valve.

When the diaphagm is pulled back the points of the contact breaker seprates and the electric to d soid is disconnected.

A spring pushes the diaphragm back to its original position and fuel in the pump is forced out, through the outlet valve to the working unit in the engine.

The pump work as the engine is inneed of fuel in the working units.

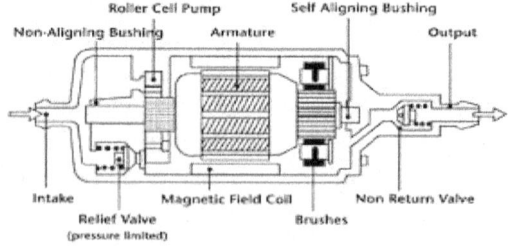

FIGURE 5.2 Electric fuel pump

5.2.4 ELECTRICAL FUEL PUMP FAULTS AND CAUSES

Pump not working	1. Check that the ignition is switch on. 2. Check circuit continuity by disconnecting the lead and check with volt meter. 3. Check that the lead to the terminal head cap is secured. 4. Examine earthing points for cleanliness 5. Examine contact point and clean, if dirty with a light wire brush. 6. Cause may be due to obstruction in suction pipe and it may be cleared by blowing air through pump intake pipe which comes from the fuel tank.
Pumps oscillates but delivers little fuel were needed	1. Choked filter or obstruction in suction side of the fuel pipe. 2. Check valve for dirt at seating flatness and wear.
pump noise	1. If the pump operates rapidly and is noisy there is probably an air leak on the suction side of the pump. Test by

	disconnecting the fuel line and immerse it in a fuel from external source and operate the pump and observe if air bubbles appear. Check all unions and joints and fuel level.

5.3 CARBURETORS

A simple carburetor only provides the correct mixture of the petrol from the tank with the right amount of air to form a spray that burns easily in the combustion chamber. A small supply of petrol from the pump is stored in the floating chamber. The position on its induction stroke draws air along the choke tube. As the air reaches the narrow part of the tube it is forced to speed up.

This increase in speed causes the pressure of the air in the venturi to fall below the pressure in the floating chamber. The difference in the two air pressure causes the petrol to flow from the floating chamber to the venturi where it is caught in the fast moving air and turned into a fine spray which is drawn into the engine. According to the direction in which the carburetor intake is located carburetors are referred to as follow.

- Downdraught
Vertical or up draught
- Side draught
- Semi-down draught

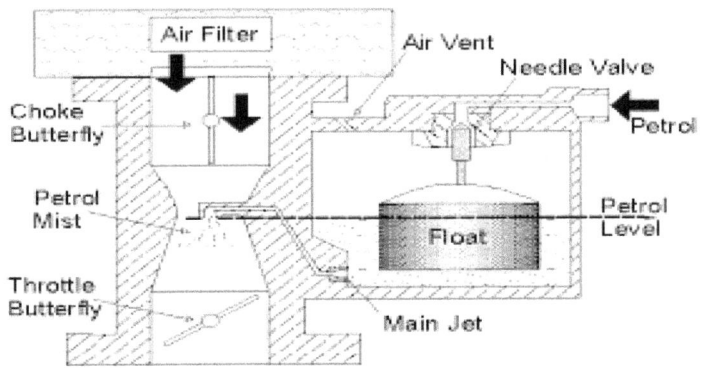

FIGURE 5.3 A carburetor

5.3.1 CARBURETOR FAULTS AND THEIR CAUSES

FAULT	CAUSES
Erratic running and stalling at idling, lucid of power high fuel consumption	Sticking piston caused by: 1. Dirty piston and suction chamber. 2. Jet out of center 3. A bent needle
Hesitation at pick-up	1. Low damper oil level requiring topping up 2. Oil with less viscosity
Float chamber flooding	1. Dirty or worn float chamber 2. Punctured float 3. Incorrect fuel level

5.4 AIR FILTER

The air drawn into the engine contains a lot of dirt and dust from the tank. This dust must not be allowed into the engine or it will cause a lot of damages to the engine. A filter is fixed to the intake of the carburetor or injector to remove the dirt. There are many types of filter, but the most common type is the paper-element, oil bath and wire-mesh.

5.5 PAPER-ELEMENT FILTER

The air is drawn through a special type of paper folded into zigzag to give a very large surface area. The dirt is left on the paper, leaving clean air to enter the engine.

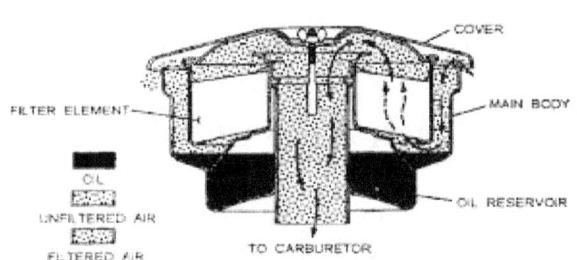

Figure 5.4 oil bath air cleaner

6.0 COMBUSTION

Combustion in compression ignition engine

In a CI engine the fuel is sprayed directly into the cylinder and the fuel-air mixture ignites spontaneously. This graph shows the fuel injection flow rate, net heat release rate and cylinder pressure for a direct injection CI engine.

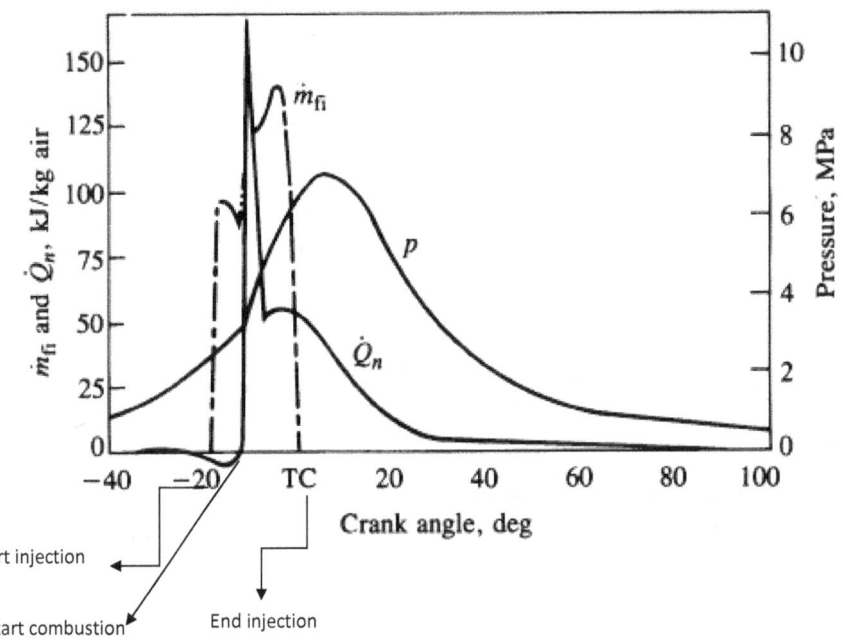

Figure 6.1 fuel injection flow rate

The combustion in ci engine is in stages which include the following:

- **Ignition delay**: - fuel is injected directly into the cylinder towards the end of the compression stroke. The liquid fuel atomizes into small drops and penetrates into the combustion chamber. The fuel vaporizes and mixes with the high temperature high-pressure air.

- **Premixed combustion phase:** – combustion of the fuel which has mixed with the air to within the flammability limits (air at high-temperature and high-pressure) during the ignition delay period occurs rapidly in a few crank angles.

- **Mixing controlled combustion phase:** – after premixed gas consumed, the burning rate is controlled by the rate at which mixture becomes available for burning. The rate of burning is controlled in this phase primarily by the fuel-air mixing process.

- **Late combustion phase:** – heat release may proceed at a lower rate well into the expansion stroke (no additional fuel injected during this phase). Combustion of any unburned liquid fuel and soot is responsible for this.

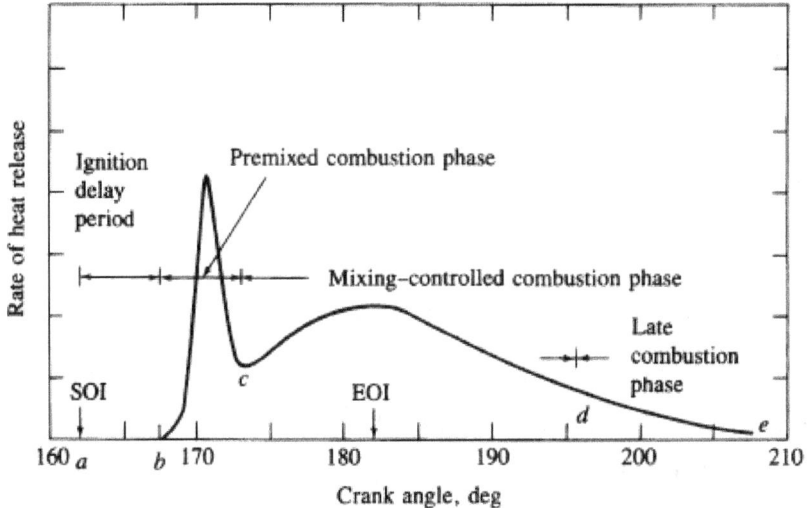

Figure 6.2 four stages of combustion in ci engine

The compression ignition engine is categorized into two types:

1. Direct injection
2. Indirect injection

1. **Direct-injection**: – have a single open head which the nozzle inject the fuel into directly into the combustion chamber. It is usually use in large stationary engine, which operates at a low speed which the time for mixing to appropriate proportion is long. So when designing a open of shallow bowl is adopted to help increase the rate of burning and engine efficiency.

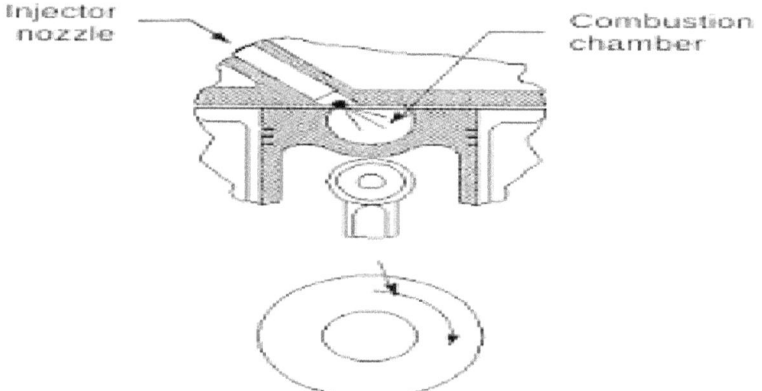

Figure 6.3 direct injection

MERIT AND DEMERIT OF DIRECT INJECTION

S/N	MERIT	DEMERIT
1	Slight lower fuel consumption due to reduced heat losses	Injection pressures are higher so wear and tear of injection equipment is higher.
2	Easier cold starting due to reduced heat losses. / No starting devices.	Injection equipment needs more frequent skilled servicing.
3	Injection pressure are relatively higher	Need good quality of fuel for good performance and clean exhaust
4	Smoother running due to highly pressure rate	To small engines, the high pressure spray is needed for atomization causes fuel to be deposited on the combustion chamber wall.

2. **Indirect-injection:** – chamber is divided into two regions and the fuel is injected into the "prechamber" which is connected to the main chamber via a nozzle, or one or more orifices. It is usually used for small high-speed engines used in automobiles chamber swirl is not sufficient, indirect injection is used where high swirl or turbulence is generated in the pre-chamber during compression and products/fuel blowdown and mix with main chamber air.

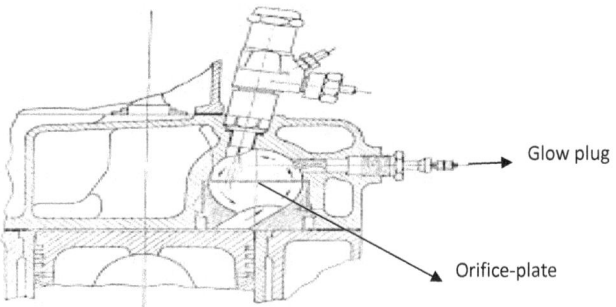

Figure 6.4 indirect injection

MERIT AND DEMERIT OF INDIRECT INJECTION

S/N	MERIT	DEMERIT
1	Less sensitive to fuel quality	Greater fuel consumption
2	Softer spray and lower wear and tear on the injection equipment	More difficult cold starting due to greater area of cold surface
3	The pintle nozzle is much less likely to become clogged or blocked than multi hole nozzle	May require cold starting aid glow plug or manifold air heater devices
4	It is suitable for small engine	Less efficient in performance

7. 0 GAS TURBINE

Gas turbine is versatile items of turbo machinery it can be used in several field of life for example power generation, aviation, marine field e.tc.

Various mechanical devices have been used to produce power for industry and society needs. Analysis on stream power plant shows that heat was added to the water and the water vapor expanded through a steam turbine, producing work. The thermal efficiency of a 500LMIN plant is about 40%. One case of the inefficiency is that an intermediate fluid, water is used to transfer the energy of the hot combustion gases to the steam turbine.

Gas turbine units overcome this by using the combustion gases directly in the turbine. A very important factor in gas-turbine selection is that gas turbine power plants are very compact and lightweight. The conventional steam power plant must occupy a far greater area and also much heavier.

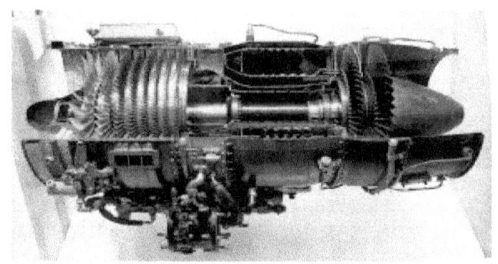

Figure 7.1 a simple gas turbine

7.1 FUNDAMENTALS OF GAS TURBINE

For a gas turbine to produce any work, in hot and low pressure. Therefore, the gases must first be compressed. If after the compression the fluid is expanded through the turbine, the power produced would be used equally by the compressor, provided that both the turbine and compressor functioned ideally. If heat is added to the fluid before it reached the turbine, raising the temperature then an increase in power output should be achieved.

Unfortunately this cannot occur, the turbine blades have a metallurgical thermal limit. If the gas enters continuously higher than the temperature, the combined thermal and material stresses on the blade will cause it to inefficiency and later fail.

Typically inlet temperatures of 1300k may be found on industrial turbines.

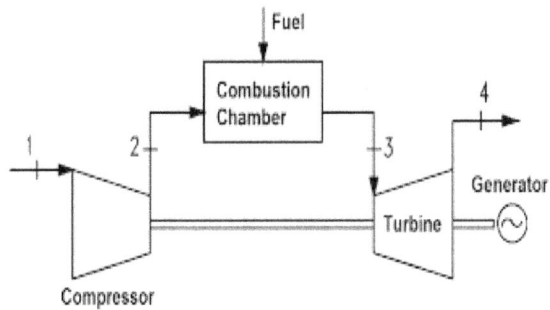

Figure 7.2 simple open cycle gas turbine

7.2 THE CYCLE ANALYSIS

The gas-turbine cycle may either be closed or open. The more common cycle is the open, in which atmospheric air is continuously drawn into the compressor, heat is added to the air by the combustion of fuel and the fluid expands through the turbine and exhausts to the atmosphere.

In the closed cycle, the heat must be added to the fluid in a nuclear power plant, and the fluid must be cooled after it leaves the turbine and before it enters the compressor.

The air-standard Brayton cycle is the ideal closed system gas-turbine cycle. It is characteristized by constant pressure heat addition and heat rejection and is entropic compression and expansion processes.

Air is the working fluid and may be considered an ideal gas. The steady-flow constant pressure processed during which heat is transferred are no longer constant temperature processes and the ideal efficiency must therefore be appreciably less than the Carnot efficiency based upon the maximum and minimum temperature of the cycle.

Also, the negative compressor work, CP (T_1-T_2) is an appreciable proportion of the positive expansion work CP (T_3-T_4), so that the work ratio is considerably less than Rankine cycle and it is much more susceptible to irreversibility.

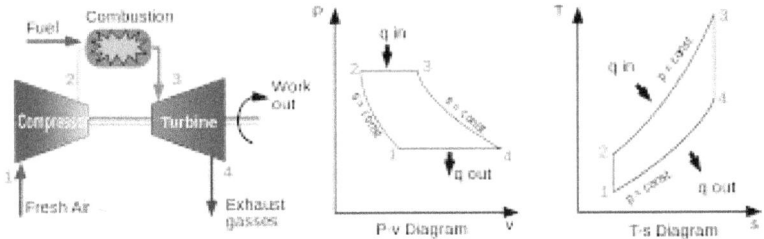

Figure 7.3 baryton cycle

The thermal efficiency 7th of the Brayton cycle may found as follows:

$7^{th} = \dfrac{Wnet}{Qin} = \dfrac{EQ}{Qin} = \dfrac{Qin-Qin}{Qin} = 1-\dfrac{Q_2}{Q_1}$

$Q_1 = mcp\,(T_3-T_2)$

$Q_2 = mcp\,(T_4-T_1)$

$7^{th} = 1-\dfrac{T_4-T_1}{T_3-T_2}$ .... equation (1)

The pressure ratio, rp is defined as:

$Rp = p_2/p_1$

And from isentropic expansion and compression processes, we find that

$\dfrac{T_2}{T_1} = \dfrac{T_3}{T_4}$

Therefore, $T_4 = \dfrac{T_3}{T_2}\,T_1$ ....equation ii

Substituting equation ii into equation i

$7^{th} = 1-\dfrac{T_3/T_2\ T_1-T_2}{T_3-T_2}$

$$7^{th} = 1 - \frac{T_1 (T_3/T_2.1)}{T_2 (T_3-1)}$$

$$7^{th} = 1 - \frac{T_1}{T_2}$$

Relating the cycle temperature to the pressure ratio

$$Tp = P_2/P_1 = P_3/P_4$$

For isentropic compression and expansion

$$\frac{T_2}{T_1} = \frac{p_2}{\{p_1\}} = rp^{\,r\text{-}1/r}$$

Or $\dfrac{T_1}{T_2} = \dfrac{1}{rp^{\,r\text{-}1/r}}$

$$7^{th} = 1 - \frac{1}{rp^{\,r\text{-}1/r}}$$

Thus, for the Brayton cycle the thermal efficiency is a function of the pressure ratio rp. The maximum temperature does have an effect on the optimum performance. If T_3 and T_1 are fixed, then there will be an optimum pressure ratio to produce a maximum amount of work, Wnet. The

Variable temperature is T_2, the temperature of the fluid leaving the compressor.

Wnet= work output from Turbine-Work input to compressor:

Work output from turbine

$$(h_3-h_4) = Cp (T_3-T_4)$$

Work input to compressor

$$(h_2-h_1) = Cp (T_2-T_1)$$

$$Wnet = Cp (T_3-T_4) - Cp (T_2-T_1)$$

But $T_4 = \dfrac{T_3.T_1}{T_2}$

$Wnet = \dfrac{Cp\ (T_3-T_3.T1-T_2+T_1)}{T_2}$

For Wnet to be maximum the $dWnet/dT_2 = 0$

$dWnet = \dfrac{Cp\ (T_3-T_3.T_1-T_2+T_1)dT_2}{T_2}$

$Cp\ \dfrac{(T_3.T_1)}{T_2^2} - 1 = 0$

$\dfrac{T_3.T_1}{T^2} = 1$

$T_2 = \sqrt{T_3.T_1}$

Work ratio $= \dfrac{Network}{Gross\ work}$

$\dfrac{Cp\ (T_3-T_4) - Cp\ (T_2-T_1)}{Cp\ (T_3-T_4)}$

$1-\dfrac{T_2-T_1}{T_3-T_4}$

$\dfrac{T_2}{T_1}=rp^{\,r-1/r} = \dfrac{T_3}{T_4}$

$T_2 = T_1{}^{rpr-1/r}$ and $T_4 = \dfrac{T_3}{rp^{r-1/r}}$

Hence, substituting

Work ratio $= \dfrac{T_1\ (rp^{r-1/r}-1)}{T_3\ [1-(1/rp^{r-1/r})]}$

Reference

1. Lyes kadem (thermodynamics) 2007
2. Fernando Salazar (internal combustion engine) 1998
3. Penrite oil company pty.ltd (guide to oil and greases) 2008
4. Automobile training board (inspect & service cooling system)
5. Applied thermal engineering (unit 5 cooling system)
6. Ujjwa k saha (IC lubricating system)
7. Prof. Dr. cem sorusbay(combustion in SI engine)
8. Pak piston industry @www. Pakpiston.com

Identifying the Role of Physical Therapy in Soft Tissue Healing

Application of Physical Therapy to Promote Recovery
from Delayed Onset Muscle Soreness

by Dr. Orson Miller DPT

DORRANCE
PUBLISHING CO
EST. 1920
PITTSBURGH, PENNSYLVANIA 15238

Dorrance Publishing Co
585 Alpha Drive
Suite 103
Pittsburgh, PA 15238
Visit our website at *www.dorrancebookstore.com*

ISBN: 978-1-6461-0469-7
eISBN: 978-1-6461-0716-2

Identifying the Role of Physical Therapy in Soft Tissue Healing

Application of Physical Therapy to Promote Recovery
from Delayed Onset Muscle Soreness

ABSTRACT

Soft tissue damage is a common type of physical injury. Some forms of soft tissue damage, such as delayed onset muscle soreness following exercise, are often identified by physicians and patients as conditions that can be managed through rest and pain medications. Management of delayed onset muscle soreness through pain medication creates risks for the patient, such as increased resistance to painkillers and the possibility of addiction to opiate-based compounds. Management of inflammation caused by delayed onset muscle soreness through administering steroidal compounds can have negative repercussions for athletes. In a critical review of the literature, this research project explores the use of physical therapy as a strategy to reduce the pain caused by delayed onset muscle soreness and promote increased healing of soft tissue injuries. The research questions are designed to explore the use of physical therapy as a healing strategy, as it is possible that physical therapy could be used to promote recovery after injury and could also be used as a treatment regime to help encourage healing following delayed onset muscle soreness. The research study uses a qualitative research design in which a grounded literature review is used to assess the available information on physical therapy and soft tissue injury to provide evidence for the use of physical therapy in naturopathic care and healing of delayed onset muscle soreness. Findings reveal that physical therapy is not likely to benefit persons who suffer delayed onset muscle soreness and have had no training in a physical therapy regime but may be beneficial for persons who have received instruction in physical therapy prior to sustaining soft tissue injury. The research is relevant to athletes who are likely to experience the same type of soft tissue injuries due to exercise routines or because previous injuries have predisposed the soft tissue to re-injury.

Table of Contents

Chapter 1:
INTRODUCTION

Physical therapy is widely used as part of healing regimes. Patients receive training and assistance in physical therapy techniques and are able to apply these techniques to recover from injury, or less frequently, disease. The benefits of physical therapy as a recovery aid are well-known and are generally accepted within the medical community as an appropriate component of health care.

The role that physical therapy plays in physiological reconstruction has been studied with less depth and frequency. While it is recognized that physical therapy affects the patient's physiological status and plays a significant role in recuperation, physical therapy is almost always relegated to a therapeutic role during the recovery process and is not considered to affect the initial healing process. As such, physical therapy tends to be integrated into a patient's healing regime only after a specific state of recovery has been attained and the patient is considered healthy enough to withstand the stress and rigors resulting from participation in physical therapy (Houglum, 1992).

Research into soft tissue wound healing indicates that soft tissue is a durable compound that responds to specific forms of stimulation (Almekinders, 1996). It has been demonstrated that the healing rate of soft tissue can be improved through massage (Houglum, 1992), compression therapy (Kraemer et al., 2001), substance application (e.g. nonsteroidal anti-inflammatory drugs or growth factor therapy) (Hom, Thatcher, & Tibesar, 2002; Dahners & Mullis, 2004), or through pulsed electrical stimulation (Gottrup, Agren, & Karlsmark, 2000). Examination of different aspects of the healing process suggests that some of these strategies may be beneficial in narrow contexts but may otherwise damage the patient's soft tissue, which has prompted researchers to caution that soft tissue healing strategies must be selectively determined on a case-by-case basis (Gottrup et al., 2000). It has also been recognized that physical therapy may have broader applications as part of the initial healing process as opposed to being limited to the recuperation phases of treatment regimens (Jette, 1995). It is possible that physical therapy might not only help patients recover from soft tissue damage after the initial injury has had some time to heal but might be used to promote healing.

Background

Soft tissue consists of connective tissues that connect or support structures and organs (Almekinders, 1996). In clinical application, the term *soft tissue* can be applied to ligaments, muscle, nerves, tendons, blood vessels, fat, fascia, and synovial tissues; health care practitioners are required to be specific concerning the type of soft tissue presenting in a given medical case. Soft tissue injuries pose challenges for health care practitioners because of their placement, as these tissues can suffer injury but are hidden underneath skin and muscle. Diagnosis of soft tissue injury can be difficult as medical imaging technologies are less likely to identify problems in soft tissue than in other sites, but improvements in imaging technologies have made it easier to develop a visible presentation of the injury *in situ*.

Models of soft tissue healing have historically taken into account the type of soft tissue that was injured, the location on the body of the injury, and the basic physiological status of the patient (Gottrup et al., 2000; Kraemer at al., 2001). Chronic soft tissue injuries, such as arthritis, are progressive throughout the patient's lifetime, while immediate or spontaneous soft tissue injury can occur as the result of an accident or as a symptom of a different physiological condition, such as delayed onset muscle soreness following prolonged exercise

(Kraemer, et al., 2001). Another type of soft tissue injury can occur within the clinical health care setting, where invasive operations involve cutting into soft tissue in order to address a more serious health concern (Gottrup, et al., 2000). As each of these conditions has a separate identifiable cause and may indicate different treatment and healing regimes, soft tissue injuries are historically identified as a general condition and progressive delimitations are applied to selectively identify how, why, and to what extent a specific injury is unique and in what respects treatment should be applied.

Medications used in the management of pain are frequently viewed as an appropriate and accurate strategy to reduce the sensations of pain. Physicians are aware of the potential negative repercussions associated with the use of pain management medications, particularly those that have addictive properties or side effects that evoke negative physiological responses in the patient (e.g. nausea). Certain categories of patients, such as children and the elderly, might suffer from psychological damage associated with long-term exposure to pain and are therefore likely to benefit from the use of pain medications as opposed to alternative therapies (Howard, 2003). However, both physicians and patients have demonstrated reluctance to rely upon pain medication as the sole means of controlling the symptoms of pain.

Physical therapy is widely recognized as a necessary component of many healing regimes. It is commonly applied to a patient following an initial re-covery period from damage or other physical injury but can also be used for patients who have physical conditions that can be positively affected through the use of physical therapy (Jette, 1995). As such, physical therapy is generally categorized as an impairment and disability treatment strategy in which mo-bility and endurance are gradually improved through long-term healing. Phys-ical therapy is traditionally delivered to a patient using session-based therapy, where meetings between the patient and the physical therapist are necessary to guide the patient through the physical routines and instruct the patient in the appropriate exercise and mobility strategies.

It has been suggested that physical therapy has broader applications than those found in treating impairment or injury (Jette, 1995). Some practitioners have suggested that physical therapy provides demonstrable outcomes in terms of promoting recovery and recommend that additional research be done to identify whether there are additional potential applications for physical therapy in the clinical setting (Jette, 1995). In a broader context, physical therapy may help facilitate healing in ways that go beyond impairment treatment and recovery.

Statement of the Problem

While physical therapy is widely used in health care as a strategy designed to promote recovery from injury, it is possible that physical therapy could be used to help promote healing in other ways. Physical healing has been applied to some types of soft tissue injury after an initial recovery period has passed, thus helping assist in recovery from injury. However, certain forms of soft tissue injuries do not require immediate surgical treatment (Almekinders, 1996). A prominent example of this type of injury is found in delayed onset muscle soreness following exercise, where a patient has caused damage to his or her soft tissue during physical activity. Patients with such injuries typically treat them through self-medication, where over-the-counter pharmaceuticals are taken to reduce the sensations of pain.

However, physical therapy may have broader applications beyond its conventional use in treating impairment and injury. It is possible that physical therapy could potentially be used to promote healing in soft tissue injuries, and in doing so, would help hasten patients' recovery from injury. Patients with delayed onset muscle soreness can potentially reduce pain and promote healing if they received training and assistance in physical therapy. The problem statement which governs the proposed research study is therefore:

Healing regimes traditionally incorporate physical therapy after an initial recovery period has reduced the traumatic effects associated with impairment or injury, but the careful and appropriate introduction of physical therapy at an earlier period in a healing regime may potentially accelerate the initial healing process.

Purpose of the Study

The purpose of the research study is to gather and provide evidence that physical therapy can be used as a component of the healing process in delayed onset muscle soreness following exercise. Traditionally, physical therapy has been used in the recovery phase after an injury has occurred and some marginal healing has taken place. Yet the type of soft tissue injury that occurs during exercise is typically extended over a muscle group instead of directly injuring a limited aspect of the muscle site as occurs during surgery or with a cutting impact injury. Delayed onset muscle soreness following exercise can be painful, but it is distinctive from other soft tissue injuries in that there is no impact injury and the injury itself is generally distributed throughout the muscle group (Almekinders, 1996). As a result, while delayed onset muscle soreness can be painful, it is distinctive from other forms of soft tissue injury because the muscle itself maintains its integrity. These characteristics have made it suitable as the type of soft tissue injury explored in the proposed study as there is less physical risk to the subjects than selecting subjects recovering from surgery or who have recently experienced an auto accident.

If it can be successfully proven that patients who receive instruction in physical therapy are able to manage their pain and promote their recovery through engaging in a specific physical therapy regime, this research study can help provide evidence that pain medications are not mandatory for the treatment of pain. The study will help demonstrate that self-care strategies that can reduce pain and help promote improved healing are possible if the patient receives instruction in appropriate techniques. These self-care strategies are valuable for those persons seeking to improve their control over soft-tissue injury or seek to prevent future injury; additionally, practitioners of the naturopathic discipline can benefit from the information contained in this study as it helps introduce information on soft-tissue injury and can provide recommendations for healing and prevention.

Rationale of the Research Project

Medication plays a prominent role in modern society. Persons engaging in physical care and self-maintenance are prone to use pharmaceuticals instead of alternative strategies to help preserve and promote their health. These conditions can result in dependence upon medications as the preferred method of self-treatment, and this perceived dependence can create subsequent problems among users. Painkiller abuse is one concern, especially with prescribed drugs, such as opioids (e.g. oxycodone and codeine). There is the growing problem where prescription painkillers are increasingly used as a recreational drug by adolescents, where the number of adolescents using marijuana has decreased significantly over the past five years, but the number of adolescents abusing prescription painkillers has risen dramatically (Bender, 2007). These findings have caused some authorities in the medical community to caution that prescription painkillers are far too accessible in the average household (Bender, 2007). The literature also suggests that many patients and physicians are resistant to the idea of using medication as the primary strategy for pain management in certain types of injury (Ward, et al., 1993; Warfield & Kahn, 1995). It is possible that through information and improving the awareness of the impact of pain medication on the patient, a transformation in thinking about the advantages of pain medication can be attained.

More importantly, the impact that medication plays within society and within medical care introduces the question of a perceived reliance of dependence on pharmaceuticals than towards other forms of self-care. Patients identify their physical status as one that can be affected by drugs as opposed to one that can be managed through other treatment strategies (Pinsky, 2004). It is important to communicate to patients that they can identify their body's needs and manage many of these without relying upon pharmaceuticals for treatment. Yet it is also likely that accomplishing this goal will require communication with the patient; such communication is intended to promote awareness and encourage the patient to adopt a new way of thinking about his or her life. The research project will seek to explore how patients who have treated delayed onset muscle soreness through the use of pain medication can be encouraged to learn physical therapy techniques and incorporate these into their health care regimes instead of relying upon medication. It is anticipated that the research project will help formulate new ideas and objectives that are associated with self-care and self-healing and that the patients can use this information to educate themselves how to prevent and treat soft-tissue injury while under the care of a competent medical care provider.

Significance of the Study

The proposed study will be significant in that it may provide alternative methods of pain management and injury recovery that do not rely upon prescription drugs to help promote healing. These conditions are especially important for persons who routinely experience delayed onset muscle soreness as part of their lifestyles; persons who are physically active often encounter soft tissue damage as a result of overextension of their muscles. Overextension has been shown to have a negative impact upon their physical health for two dissimilar reasons; many athletes choose to push themselves beyond the limits of endurance in the belief that such behaviors help improve conditioning and some persons who are new to physical exercise may be dissuaded from continuing if they experience pain and soreness (Bender, 2007). As a result, many persons who experience delayed onset muscle soreness may engage in treatment strategies that do not effectively target the problem but instead can compromise their long-term health.

The proposed study is significant in that it promotes an alternative strategy to healing that encourages physical movement. While physical therapy is not exercise and should not be considered as such, it does enable continued physical movement, even when the affected person is no longer able to maintain his or her normal physical routine (Almekinders, 1996). If persons who experience delayed onset muscle soreness are encouraged to think of physical therapy after they have experienced soft tissue injury, they can still engage in muscle movement and maintain limited activity during the healing process. Doing so may promote mobility and encourage stability within the routines of persons who wish to engage in physical activity.

The study is significant in that it also encourages alternative thinking towards pain management strategies in which medication is minimized. Modern health care emphasizes pain medication as a component of recovery regimes as it helps alleviate the psychological stress associated with physical injury (Almekinders, 1996). For persons who experience delayed onset muscle soreness, it may be possible to encourage healing and therapy regimes through the promotion of physical therapy; while there is pain associated with physical therapy, when performed correctly, the patient regains mobility, flexibility, and reduces the symptoms associated with the original injury. Finally, after the initial instruction period during which the patient receives training in physical therapy, the patient can engage in physical therapy independent of supervision. The patient will save money on pain medications and their potential side effects, and on consultations with health care professionals, which in turn will also allow the health care industry to save money from continuous treatment of the same problems. As such, if it is proven that physical therapy helps to alleviate pain after delayed onset muscle soreness following exercise; it can be recommended as an advantageous strategy for healing and health care.

Research Questions

Three research questions are used to guide this research study. These are stated as follows:

1. What is the role of physical therapy in soft tissue healing?
2. What is the impact of physical therapy on delayed onset muscle soreness?
3. Does instruction in physical therapy help persons suffering from delayed onset muscle soreness manage pain?

CHAPTER II:
LITERATURE REVIEW

The literature review addresses the information in the subject areas first posed to the readers in the Introduction. This literature review is organized according to theme and addresses the main concepts introduced in the preceding section. The information contained herein will require expansion for the finished dissertation but is presented to demonstrate the type of research being conducted and the themes that are used to organize the information.

Pain Management

Pain management in the clinical care setting has traditionally been dominated by the use of pharmacological substances designed to alter the patient's perception of pain. In terms of physiological impact on the body, pain is identified as "the acute activation of small sensory afferent axons by high intensity thermal and mechanical stimuli [which] evokes locally organized spinal motor reflexes (nociceptive reflexes), autonomic responses, and pain behavior" (Warfield & Bajwa, 2004, p. 13). The persistence of these responses is determined by the severity of the injury, resulting in continuing stimuli that serves to evoke a persistent, and often, worsening sensation of pain in the affected person. When pain management is introduced, the effect of these stimuli "is mediated by the local encoding of afferent input at the level of the dorsal horn and the activation of spinofugal projection neurons" (Warfield & Bajwa, 2004,

p. 13). The reflex actions associated with pain are suppressed, resulting in a reduction in pain. Physicians and health care specialists who are active with patients who suffer from pain are typically certified by the American Board of Anesthesiology (ABA) and have completed a fellowship in pain management (Abram, 2004). It is believed that this additional training in pain management will ensure that the physician or specialist has received a sufficient background in pain management and will have the information required to prescribe the appropriate medication for the patient's condition, if medication is required. Pain management training is also used to help the physician or specialist in the diagnosis of pain, which is a complicated and frequently inaccurate stage of patient care (Wolff, 2005). Indeed, while significant advances have been made in the 20th century in the diagnosis and the assessment of pain, "we still lack a generally accepted definition of pain" (Wolff, 2005, 4). According to Wolff (2005):

Both clinically and in the laboratory, pain tends to be defined operationally, such as withdrawal from a noxious stimulus, the patient or subject saying "pain," marking a point along a line, relaxing tense muscles. However, pain defined in this manner can strictly speaking only refer to the specific situation rather than act as an absolute. Consequently, it is yet premature to define pain in absolute terms (p. 4).

Those involved in pain management are thus hard-pressed to attach precise assessments of pain to patients, as they lack not only a working definition of pain, but the sensation of pain differs on a case-by-case basis. Efforts to provide functional pain management standards are ongoing, and these standards show distinction among types of pain and efforts to clarify how, why, and to what extent pain affects patients (Phillips, 2000). These standards, unfortunately, still cannot provide a functional assessment of all instances of pain and must still be interpreted through ongoing communication between the patient and the patient's medical team (Phillips, 2000). Treatment for chronic pain is further complicated through the patient's response to early pain management regimes used in their treatment. Pain management is therefore best understood as an ongoing process; moreover it is an extremely complex process that requires ongoing input from both the patient and the physician to explore the patient's past medical history and to identify the patient's current psycho-logical and psychological state.

The most effective and quickest-acting strategy used to target the reflex actions that cause pain is through the use of medication. Pain medication causes an analgesic response in the patient, which does not treat the causes of pain but does reduce the impact of the symptoms that cause a pain response in patients. Pain management drugs act primarily on the central nervous sys-tem (CNS) and on the peripheral nervous system (PNS). The type of analgesic response that affects the patient is determined by the drug used, and while cer-tain categories of pain medication have proven effective in the management of certain types of pain, the effectiveness of various pain medication changes based upon the needs and responsiveness of individual patients. The category of pain medications that has proven almost universally effective in managing pain are naturally-occurring narcotics, such as morphine or synthetic narcotics. Unfortunately, the advantages of the effectiveness of these drugs are mitigated by their addictive properties, as the physiological impact of narcotics not only relieves pain but causes dependency in the majority of patients who use them for a prolonged period.

Drugs that are not narcotics also have potent side effects, many of these causing new or distinctive forms of pain in their own right. Potent psychotro-pic drugs may be used to treat both acute and chronic pain but are also likely to cause nausea and other forms of physical discomfort. For patients with chronic pain, long-term exposure to these drugs can cause symptoms, such as physical exhaustion, and has been correlated with psychological side effects, such as depression. It has been noted that treatment of chronic pain using pain medication is merely a process of trading one disabling condition for another.

Physicians' Attitudes Towards Pain Management

Physicians' attitudes towards pain vary widely and patients who suffer from chronic pain often seek to align themselves with a physician whose attitudes are in keeping with their own. For physicians and specialists who work closely with patients who suffer from chronic pain caused by debilitating diseases or disorders (e.g. cancer), acceptance of the use of pain medication increases (Von Roenn, Cleeland, Gonin, Hatfield & Pandya, 1993). Physicians and specialists who work with patients who suffer intense acute pain (e.g. broken bones, childbirth, etc.) typically accept the necessity of pain medication to treat both the immediate pain that follows the initial incident and to manage the pain as the injury heals.

However, physicians and specialists who work with patients who suffer from chronic pain that is not associated with a progressive disease have differing opinions concerning the appropriateness of pain management. Therapeutic pain management is increasingly popular among physicians and specialists who strive to improve the overall quality of life for patients who suffer from chronic pain that is not associated with a chronic illness. In some instances, physicians and specialists have identified pain as a result of a chronic disability as manageable through therapy. Therapeutic intervention has also been recognized as a valid strategy to promote immediate pain management while helping the patient learn how to control the conditions associated with pain and to prevent future injury (Loisel, et al., 1997).

Physicians' attitudes towards pain management also take into account the status of the patient. Physicians appear more tolerant of pain medications towards patients who are unable to manage their pain through alternative options, such as young children and the elderly (Howard, 2003). The quality-of-life experienced by the patient is taken into account during the assessment process and weighed against the patient's ability to practice alternative pain management strategies. For example, Howard (2003) recognizes that while children might be especially susceptible to the ill effects of pain management medications due to their size and developing physiology, "the experience of pain in early life may lead to long-term consequences" (p. 2464). Similarly, patients who are elderly and suffer from dementia and other cognitive disorders might not be able to comprehend why the negative sensations of pain occur and might be unable to successfully participate in alternative pain management strategies. Physicians therefore take into consideration the psychological status of the patient in addition to their physiological condition when determining the appropriateness of pain management through medication.

Patients' Attitudes Towards Pain Management

Patients' attitudes towards pain management are similar to those held by physicians in respect to personal distinctions concerning pain, affecting the perceptions of appropriate pain management. Adults surveyed on the topic of pain management and its impact on their overall physical health often report that the advantages of pain medication are outweighed by its disadvantages (Warfield & Kahn, 1996). Intriguingly, research into pain management has shown that many patients would prefer to manage their pain without the use of medication. In an early study into how cancer patients perceive pain medication and its impact on their lives, 85% of patients reported that they had concerns over how pain medication affected them, and 35% reported that they would not use pain medication if alternatives were available to them. The researchers did add to caveats, where "Those who were older, less educated, or had lower incomes were more likely to have concerns [and] higher levels of concern were correlated with higher levels of pain" (Ward et al., 1993, p. 319). The researchers suggested that a lack of education or information concerning the impact of pain management on the person leads to the confusion over the appropriateness of using pain medication. If this is the case, then the patient is more likely to resist receiving pain medication as part of the treatment regime. However, the researchers also found that patients who had progressively worsening cancer and who received pain medication were also more resistant to its use, suggesting that continued exposure to high doses of pain management medications had an impact on the patients' willingness to use it. The researchers concluded that patients who received high doses of pain management medication suffered from side effects associated with the drugs and wished to avoid these if possible.

Therapists' Attitudes towards Pain Management

Clinical pain management is a complex process and differs according to the clinician's specialty and the characteristics of the patient's unique case history. Therapists' attitudes towards pain management differ according to these conditions, as the practicing therapist is aware that pain is an experiential condition

and cannot be generalized by either the health care professional or by the af-
flicted patient. To help clarify how therapists perceive pain management, assessment of health care professionals' attitudes towards pain management tends
to apply categories of pain, pain management, and clinical experience to help
clarify how health care specialists approach clinical pain management. For example, Clarke, French, Bilodeau, and Capasso (1996) explored "nurses' characteristics, including previous pain education, clinical experience, area of clinical
practice, and other variables and knowledge, attitudes, and clinical practice" (p.
18). These "attitudes" were applicable to specific areas of patient care, including
"non-pharmacological interventions to relieve pain, the difference between
acute and chronic pain, and the anatomy and physiology of pain" (p. 18).

When health care professionals from different clinical disciplines are con-
sulted, their attitudes towards pain and pain management suggest different
opinions of pain and how pain should be managed. Lebovits, et al. (1997), surveyed a total of "86 nurses, physicians, pharmacists, and medical/nursing stu-
dents from three hospitals" to compare and contrast the differences of medical
professionals from different specialties on their "knowledge and beliefs about
pain" (p. 237). The researchers found that physicians demonstrated the greatest informed knowledge concerning pain management, which suggested that
they were able to apply education and training in pain management to their
patients. Nurses and pharmacists, who had not received specialized education
and training in pain management, had significantly lower scores when compared to physicians. Anesthesiologists and others specializing in pain management demonstrated greater overall awareness of pain and pain management
strategies, while surgeons had lower overall scores. The researchers concluded
that health care professionals who worked with patients experiencing pain were
most likely to know how to manage pain and were more likely to develop a
patient care regime that took a patient's unique pain considerations into account. However, they also noted that many health care professionals appeared
to have "significant knowledge deficits regarding currently accepted principles
of pain management practice" and that these knowledge deficits as well as beliefs that could interfere with optimal care" are restricting patients' access to
appropriate pain management strategies (p. 237).

Physical therapists have alternately been categorized as part of both conventional and alternative medical practice (Haetzman, Elliott, Smith, Hannaford, & Chambers, 2003). Physical therapists engage with patients directly and are traditionally unable to prescribe medication, although they frequently work with physicians who can. The physical therapist recognized that pain management is part of the rehabilitation process, as repairing damage to the patient's physiological status requires physical conditioning and this conditioning is likely to place the patient at risk for experiencing pain (Haetzman, et al., 2003). Beyond these commonly-held assumptions towards pain and pain management, physical therapists do not share a single opinion towards how pain should be managed and often adapt their recommendations for pain management based on the individual case history of the patient (Haetzman, et al., 2003; Wolff, 2005).

Pain Management and Addiction to Medication

Addiction to medication is a "chronic, relapsing disease that results from the prolonged effects of drugs on the brain" (Leshner, 2003, p. 190). When identified as a brain disease, "addiction has embedded behavioral and social-context aspects that are important parts of the disorder itself" (Leshner, 2003, p. 190). Treatment of addiction is a demanding, resource-intensive procedure and the addict might suffer from the symptoms of drug addiction throughout his or her lifetime.

When prescribing medications, physicians and health care practitioners strive to be aware of any potentially addictive properties associated with a specific pharmacological substance. Unfortunately, the majority of medications prescribed for pain associated with soft tissue injury function through influencing the body's production of dopamine; this is especially true with pharmacological substances from the opioid category (Cami & Farre, 2003). The physiological and psychological impact of opioids is widely recognized as addictive, as these substances not only reduce the perception of pain but also increase production of dopamine, a hormone that has been associated to sensations of physical satisfaction and the gratification of needs (Cami & Farre,

2003). The cyclooxygenase-2 (COX-2) inhibitors are a comparatively new class of medication that shows potential in pain management, but there is a growing body of evidence to suggest that this class of medications might have a negative impact on the healing process (Seidenberg & An, 2003).

The management of temporary and chronic pain requires different strategies and different medications (Smith, Audette & Royal, 2002; Gourlay, Heit, & Almahrezi, 2005). While opioids have generally been avoided in all but the worst cases requiring potent pain management, some researchers have suggested that opioids can be successfully used to treat lesser pain as long as precautions to prevent addiction are taken (Gourlay et al., 2005). Other researchers, however, have noted that the effectiveness of opioids does not offset the detrimental aspects associated with their use, addiction being one of the most prominent examples of same (Smith et al., 2002; Pinsky, 2004). This is especially true in cases where pain is recurring; patients with chronic pain who continuously rely upon opioids for management purposes are more likely to develop an addiction than patients who have suffered from a treatable injury.

Researchers and medical personnel who work with patients with acute and chronic soft tissue injury are aware of the risks associated with the pharmacological management of pain. Nadler (2004) notes that "pain is a complex phenomenon with various causes and issues associated with its occurrence" and that pharmacological management of pain is an oversimplification of the treatment strategies available (p. 6). Also, some of the treatment strategies that are traditionally used to help alleviate pain are only conditionally effective and might serve to exacerbate the conditions that cause pain and require medication (these points will be discussed in detail in the following sections) (Seidenberg & An, 2003; Nadler, 2004).

Soft Tissue Injury and Pain

Soft tissue injuries are recognized as a painful physiological ailment (Almekinders, 1996). The pain associated with soft tissue injury can become exacerbated over time if the injury is localized to the muscles of an area that is frequently used, such as the legs or the back. Pain can also be tangentially associated to soft tissue injury; for example, neuropathic pain and central pain have different definitions and diagnoses, and neither are the direct result of soft tissue injury, but both can be associated with the site of soft tissue injury (Scadding, 1992). The type of pain that is most frequently cited as the symptom of soft tissue injury is acute pain, which is defined as "the normal physiologic response to a noxious chemical, thermal, or mechanical stimulus, and it usually is time limited" (Nadler, 2004). The pain response to soft tissue injury is determined by the type of injury and the patient's independent pain response mechanisms; some patients have a high degree of pain tolerance and can self-diagnose their pain as manageable, while other patients with similar injuries will require assistance in pain management (Nadler, 2004).

Reoccurring pain has also been associated with soft tissue injuries. Some forms of soft tissue injuries appear subject to relapse, in which the pain subsides and the injury appears to have healed but returns after the site of the injury is provoked (Almekinders, 1996; Wallis, B. J., Lord, S. M., Barnsley, L, & Bogduk, N, 1996; Bassewitz & Shapiro, 1997). Whiplash is often identified as "chronic whiplash" for this reason, as in circumstances where the initial injury appears to have healed, symptoms associated with the original injury can emerge over the lifetime of the patient (Wallis et al., 1996, p. 804). Bassewitz and Shapiro (1997) suggest that if the site of the soft tissue injury is properly treated, the pain associated with the injury will fade within six weeks. If the pain persists beyond this point, it is an indication of additional problems that require medical attention. Bassewitz and Shapiro indicated that the implications of persistent pain associated with soft tissue injury are serious; not only does persistent pain suggest that the injury was not effectively treated, but the majority of forms of soft tissue injury are not associated with chronic pain and persistence suggests that the symptoms may become chronic. Moreover, persistent pain after the injury has been treated indicates that there might be mechanisms of the injury that were not identified during the initial treatment process. If the original injury appears to have healed successfully, but there are reoccurring pain flare-ups—referred to as *subsets*—when the original site of the injury is provoked, then it is likely that the original injury is still present in some form.

Some researchers have noted that administering some forms of pain management medication to patients suffering specific types of soft tissue injury might have an "inhibitory effect" on the recovery status of the patient (Seidenberg & An, 2003, p. 151). The use of COX-2 inhibitors in treating pain and inflammation associated with "fractures, cementless total joint replacements, soft tissue healing to bone, and spinal fusion surgeries" has been linked to slower healing rates in these patients (Seidenberg & An, 2003, p. 151). It is not specifically known at this time whether the COX-2 inhibitors actually do reduce healing and recovery rates in patients, but the early emerging evidence indicates that this may indeed be the case.

Soft Tissue Injury and Traditional Treatment Strategies

The treatment strategies that are traditionally recommended for soft tissue injury depend in large part upon the type and the site of injury (Almekinders, 1996; Kannus, 2000; Motamedi, 2003). In addition to pain and anti-inflammatory medications, the treatment strategies that are most frequently used are immobilization or compression of the site, the application of temperature, or the application of topical ointments. The majority of treatment for soft tissue injury is derived from the PRICES procedure, which refers to "protection, rest, ice, compression, elevation, and support" (Kannus, 2000, p. 55).

Minimal non-invasive cryotherapy is frequently used for soft tissue injury. The patient is required to apply ice or other forms of temperature-controlling mechanisms to the site, which acts as an anti-inflammatory agent. Typically, cryotherapy is associated with exposing the site of the injury to ice or a cold compress but can also refer to immersion in cold water (Bleakley, McDonough, & MacAuley, 2004). While cryotherapy does reduce inflammation and can temporarily improve mobility in sites surrounding soft tissue injury, it is not fully known whether cryotherapy is effective in promoting healing (Bleakley, et al., 2004; Hummard & Denegar, 2004). Some researchers have suggested that cryotherapy promotes the impression of healing, where the injury appears to regain functionality and is less painful to the patient but that these outcomes might be merely an alleviation of the primary symptoms and should not be confused with actual soft tissue healing (Bleakley, et al., 2004; Hummard & Denegar, 2004).

Immobilization is another form of treatment that has proven conditionally effective, but some physicians and researchers caution that its benefits might not outweigh its negative effect on the body. Immobilization is one of the oldest forms of treatment for soft tissue injuries, where:

Immobilization has been used for thousands of years to treat injuries to the human body. Unfortunately, immobilization may lead to deleterious effects that may compromise treatment outcome, such as muscle fiber atrophy, decreased proprioception, and loss of cervical and lumbar range of motion (ROM). This loss may be a clinically significant problem in an individual who already has compromised muscle function (Nadler, 2004; p. 7).

The successful application of immobilization of the injury depends in large part upon the site of the injury and is accomplished through multiple immobilization tools, such as support structures (e.g. braces or bandages), or for serious injury, through bed rest (Almekinders, 1996; Kannus, 2000). The latter is particularly true for soft tissue injury that was sustained through concussive force and resulted in puncture wounds or internal damage (Motamedi, 2003). Bed rest is used for patients who have experienced "neck and low back pain and associated disorders," but its use is questionable for such patients because bed rest therapy "is without any significant scientific merit. Bed rest supports immobilization with its deleterious effects on bone, connective tissue, muscle, and psychosocial well-being" (Nadler, 2004, p. 7). Research into management of soft tissue injuries that are most often treated through bracing, such as whiplash injury, cervical radiculopathy, and lumbar injuries suggests that bracing and immobilization does not provide any significant benefits in improved pain management or improved healing and recovery (Nadler, 2004).

In some instances of soft tissue injury, surgery is required (Almekinders, 1996; Motamedi, 2003). Many physicians are reluctant to use surgery to treat patients who are also athletes, as there are increased complications connected to the use of surgery when compared to the other forms of traditional treatment (Almekinders, 1996; Kannus, 2000; Motamedi, 2003). However, surgery might be the only way to successfully repair certain forms of soft tissue injury (Motamedi, 2003). It has also been noted that as surgical options and techniques increase, the complications associated with surgery are reduced, although surgery has not yet reached a stage in which all surgeries are guaranteed to return patients their full range of mobility and provide the patient a pain-free recovery (Almekinders, 1996). Patients who receive surgical treatment are likely to receive medication to help manage the pain associated with the initial injury and with the surgical repairs (Smith, Audette, & Royal, 2002).

Stevens et al. (2005) notes that soft tissue injury can be associated with soft tissue infection, especially if the skin barrier has been broken. Infection can also occur in circumstances where the injury has become inflamed through other physical ailments within the body. The researchers note that all practitioners who work with patients who have soft tissue injuries should be aware of the risk of infection, even if the skin barrier has not been broken, and suggests that early diagnosis be accomplished through monitoring the patient for one or more symptoms that are associated with infection. These are:

signs and symptoms of systemic toxicity (e.g., fever or hypothermia, tachycardia [heart rate, >100 beats/min], and hypotension [systolic blood pressure, <90 mm Hg or 20 mm Hg below baseline]) have blood drawn to determine the following laboratory parameters: results of blood culture and drug susceptibility tests, complete blood cell count with differential, and creatinine, bicarbonate, creatine phosphokinase, and C-reactive protein levels. In patients with hypotension and/or an elevated creatinine level, low serum bicarbonate level, elevated creatine phosphokinase level (2-3 times the upper limit of normal), marked left shift, or a C-reactive protein level >13 mg/L, hospitalization should be considered and a definitive etiologic diagnosis pursued aggressively by means of procedures such as Gram stain and culture of needle aspiration or punch biopsy specimens, as well as requests for a surgical consultation for inspection, exploration, and/or drainage (Stevens, 2005, p. 1374).

Furthermore, the researchers caution that even under continuous supervision that infection might emerge undetected within soft tissue injuries. There are seven additional clues to diagnosis of "potentially severe deep soft-tissue infection," which are "(1) pain disproportionate to the physical findings, (2) violaceous bullae, (3) cutaneous hemorrhage, (4) skin sloughing, (5) skin anesthesia, (6) rapid progression, and (7) gas in the tissue" (Stevens, 2005, p. 1374). If these symptoms are present, however, it might be too late to help provide effective treatment and reduce the impact of infection.

"Unfortunately, these signs and symptoms often appear later in the course of necrotizing infections. In these cases, emergent surgical evaluation is of paramount importance for both diagnostic and therapeutic reasons" (Stevens, 2005, p. 1375). As such the authors recommend due diligence for all soft tissue injuries, especially if the skin barrier has been broken.

Soft Tissue Injury and Alternative Forms of Treatment

Manipulation and mobilization of soft tissue injuries are increasingly used "in the treatment of patients with neck pain and associated disorders" (Nadler, 2004, p. 8). Strategies that promote soft tissue rehabilitation are varied and depend on the type of soft tissue and the nature of the manipulation and mobilization techniques that are deemed appropriate to the injury:

Many different types of manual treatment exist, including soft tissue myofascial release, muscle energy/contract-relax, and high-velocity low-amplitude manipulation. Soft tissue myofascial release may include various techniques, including effleurage, pétrissage, friction, and tapotement. It has been shown to improve flexibility, decrease the perception of pain, and decrease the levels of stress hormones (Nadler, 2004, p. 8).

The researcher also argues that forms of manipulation and mobilization can range from massage to "high-velocity, low-amplitude manipulative techniques" designed to force the injured soft tissue to recognize mobility demands (Nadler, 2004, p. 9). Massage, while not a traditional form of treatment for soft tissue damage, has frequently been recommended as a treatment strategy and is often incorporated into chiropractic treatment regimes.

Similarly, research is emerging in the area of early mobilization or "early, controlled mobilization" (Kannus, 2000). Early mobilization is derived from the literature and research on soft tissue back injuries, which are difficult to control through traditional immobilization procedures. Instead of immobilizing these sites, an alternative strategy of limited movement is introduced in three steps. First, "during the first one to three weeks after the injury, immobilization of the injured tissue areas allows healing without extensive scarring. [Then,] when soft-tissue regeneration begins, controlled mobilization and stretching of muscle and tendons stimulate healing. [Finally], at six to eight weeks post-injury, the rehabilitative goal is full return to pre-injury level of activity" (Kannus, 2000, p. 55). It has been suggested that these early mobilization strategies are more effective for a patient as they do not impose restrictions upon movement but instead retrain the patient in how to move without exacerbating the injury; moreover permitting limited movement helps the muscles maintain mobility throughout the recovery period (Kannus, 2000).

Researchers who work with patients who have soft tissue injuries have noted that there may be other options for pain management, such as injecting the site with botulinium toxin (Smith, et al., 2002). Botulinium toxin has a paralytic effect upon nerves and soft tissue and "is approved for the treatment of muscle overactivity associated with several disorders, such as dystonias" (Smith, et al., 2002, p. 147). Also, it has been noted that "botulinum toxin therapy may be particularly useful in soft-tissue syndromes that are refractory to traditional treatment with physical therapy, electrical muscle stimulation, and other approaches" (Smith, et al., 2002, p. 147). While research is ongoing in the application of botulinium toxin, it is possible that this might serve as a supplemental element to therapy and could be used to lessen pain during the rehabilitation process (Smith, et al., 2002). However, the researchers do caution that the use of this particular type of toxin might be limited to a narrow range of soft tissue injuries and is not universally applicable (Smith, et al., 2002).

Summary

The strategies used to treat soft tissue injuries are complex and depend upon the type of injury and its severity. Complications, such as infection or reoccurring subsets of the initial injury, can reoccur after the initial injury appears to be healed. The treatment strategies that are traditionally used to manage soft tissue injuries have been disputed in terms of effectiveness; moreover some traditional treatment strategies have been questioned in terms of their actual benefits to the patient. Some forms of alternative treatment, such as manipulation and mobilization, are used to help the patient in both healing and pain management.

CHAPTER III:
METHODOLOGY

A grounded research methodology has been proposed for this research study. Grounded literature reviews were first introduced by Glaser and Strauss in 1967 as a means of exploring existing literature for new content and information. Grounded literature reviews are a form of qualitative review in which the literature is identified according to theme and content. The information is then selected from the literature and restructured in an accessible format. The purpose of reorganization of the literature is to make it more accessible to the audience as the majority of grounded research methods are used to explore existing concepts and promote information and awareness of specific components of the same (Glaser, 1998).

Restatement of the Research Questions

The following research questions have been developed to guide the research study:

1. What is the role of physical therapy in soft tissue healing?
2. What is the impact of physical therapy on delayed onset muscle soreness?
3. Does instruction in physical therapy help persons suffering from delayed onset muscle soreness manage their pain?

Rationale of the Research Method

The grounded research methodology was selected as the best applicable strategy to explore existing literature on soft tissue injury and physical therapy. There is a significant quantity of information available on these two topics and there is also significant crossover between them in respect to healing and recovery following specific forms of injury. Addressing this information through the use of a grounded literature review will help demonstrate that these two concepts share thematic similarities and that there may be conceptual information shared between them that can be transposed to the research study. This information will help illustrate that it is possible to integrate physical therapy into the treatment of delayed onset muscle soreness in order to promote healing and minimize the use of pain medications.

Data Collection

In order to successfully conduct a grounded literature review, it is necessary to consult academic literature. Journals will be the primary source of literature for the proposed study, although these will be supplemented through non-academic sources such as popular textbooks and guides that describe common methods of care for muscle soreness and soft tissue injury. All journal articles will be acquired through the library's catalogued article files, which include both printed and digital texts.

Also, information in the academic publications may be used to expand the initial study parameters. In the initial phases of data collection for this research pre-proposal, it was found that there is new research into recommended strategies used to manage soft tissue injury. While the current policy in the medical community is to use anti-inflammatory medication and inactivity to treat muscle soreness, there is emerging research that suggests inflammation should be allowed to run its course and that muscle healing could be prompted through introducing limited mobility. More information is required on these two areas of research as these seem to be ideally suited to the purpose of the current study and would provide support for the idea that physical therapy can be used to treat delayed onset muscle soreness.

Limitations

The most pressing concern associated with the use of a grounded literature review as the primary research methodology is the acquisition of material to be assessed during the literature review. As noted the study of physical therapy as having a direct quantifiable impact upon a patient's soft tissue injury is a comparatively new topic of interest. As such, acquiring literature that is of high methodological quality might pose a problem during the results phase of the research study. As the goal of the paper is to create recommendations and evidence-based guidelines to assist naturopathic practitioners and their patients, the lack of information might pose problems.

CHAPTER IV:
RESULTS

Soft tissue damage as managed by physical therapy typically involves pain as the muscles experience regeneration during the healing process. As noted in the Literature Review, physical therapists do not share a single opinion of how pain should be managed and are willing to adapt their perceptions of appropriate pain management by evaluating the needs of the individual patient. Physical therapy as a means of treating soft tissue damage is approached on a case-by-case basis to identify the needs of the patient and the strategies that can be best applied to help manage pain and to help enhance the recovery process. In the past, physical therapy has also been identified as both a conventional and an alternative therapy, although physical therapy has become widely accepted as a necessary part of conventional therapy in rehabilitation after injury (Dillin & Slabaugh, 1986; Haetzman et al., 2003).

This chapter will explore the literature on soft tissue damage and how it responds to physical therapy, especially soft tissue damage induced by exercise or sports injuries. Through exploring the literature on soft tissue injury and delayed onset muscle soreness, this chapter will provide evidence about the impact that physical therapy has on the recovery process. Information on the management of soft tissue injury will also include how pharmaceuticals are applied, such as anti-infection agents, tissue rebuilding agents, and pain medication.

Physical Therapy and its Impact on Soft Tissue Healing

All soft tissue injury is complex (Houghlum, 1992). The composition of soft tissue is such that realignment of tissue or muscle fibers is not a simple process of reconstituting the existing structure, as occurs in injury to bone. Rather, the site of injury and the type of soft tissue injured has specific requirements that for healing (Chaitow, 1987). However, these requirements can be advantageous in some circumstances, as soft tissue injury can be positively affected by intervention strategies.

Physical therapy is an intervention strategy that is designed to promote the long-term health and recovery of soft tissue. Manipulation of soft tissue through physical therapy is often mistakenly assumed to promote recovery by "curing" the injury, but this is not the case. When damage to soft tissue occurs, the soft tissue suffers impairment. The impairment limits how the soft tissue is able to perform when called on to complete specific tasks; if left to heal without intervention, the soft tissue might recover, but the impairment might persist. Again, the ambiguity in these statements is because soft tissue injury differs on a case-by-case basis and one patient's physiological response to soft tissue injury might be extremely different from those experienced by a different patient who has the same type of injury.

Some localized soft tissue injuries demonstrate improved overall recovery if the patient receives physical therapy. The purpose of physical therapy is to return the soft tissue to a state where the soft tissue is able to function in a normal manner or as close to normal as possible considering the severity of the injury (Radomski & Trombly, 2008). Herring (1990) stated that there are five specific goals of the physical therapy process: (1) establishment of an accurate diagnosis; (2) minimization of deleterious local effects of the acute injury; (3) allowance for proper healing; (4) maintenance of other components of athletic fitness; and (5) return to normal athletic function (p. 453). Of these an accurate diagnosis might be the most important and most understated aspect of the physical therapy process (Herring, 1990). Many soft tissue injuries are grouped together in the diagnosis process, such as referring to all injuries sustained in a single event as the result of concussive force rather than distinguishing them according to the type of injury, however, determining the nature of injury and administering an accurate diagnosis will ensure that the patient receives physical therapy that is appropriate to the injury.

When the patient receives physical therapy, the therapist considered the damage to the soft tissue and provides a prognosis for the patient based on the time, effort, and level of activity that the patient puts into physical therapy (Chaitow, 1987; Radomski & Trombly, 2008). Over time the damage to the soft tissue can be influenced to improve the patient's recovery, but this is done with appreciation for physical therapy as a process that can take place over weeks, months, or even years.

Whether physical therapy can actually promote the immediate healing process is, however, a different issue altogether. There is evidence that mobility and muscle use can promote the stability of soft tissue in muscles, and new research indicates that physical therapy can influences the processes of healing. The physical composition of the soft tissue is also of interest, as researchers are learning that issues such as fat content or low calcium influence the healing process. The literature on these issues will be examined in the following section.

Soft Tissue Modification through Physical Therapy

The data is inconclusive with respect to how physical therapy influences the healing process. What is better understood is how physical therapy can be used to modify soft tissue and improve development. Research in soft tissue modification is frequently done on infants and young children who are at high risk for developmental handicaps, and the influences of physical therapy are used to show how soft tissue manipulation can prevent the onset of serious complications as the result of a progressive disease. Piper et al. (1986) initially proposed that infants who were at high risk for developing neurological sequelae could be given preventative treatment through physical therapy. The researchers hypothesized that treatment would encourage normal neuromuscular development and reduce the infants' risk of manifesting the disease. The infants received physical therapy for 12 months following birth. Unfortunately, the researchers concluded that there were no substantial differences between the physiological status of the infants in the experimental and the control groups.

Despite the failure of Piper et al. (1986) to produce positive results, on-going research in preventative pediatric physical therapy has suggested that physical therapy does have beneficial outcomes when used to remodel soft tissue and prevent future soft tissue disorders. In a clinical trial, Mayo (1991) assessed the application of physical therapy on infants and young children who were under 18 months of age and who had been diagnosed with cerebral palsy. The researcher theorized that a physical therapy regime had shown beneficial effects on persons with cerebral palsy and that these effects might be realized if the regime was intensified and was delivered to infants who were at high risk for developing cerebral palsy but did not demonstrate any symptoms except for motor delay. The researcher tested her theory on 17 infants who had shown motor delay and administered a physical therapy regime in which the infants received physical therapy on a weekly basis. When contrasted to infants who received physical therapy on a monthly regime, the results clearly demonstrated an improvement in neurological and muscular development. The researcher concluded that physical therapy had the potential to remodel soft tissue in infants and could be used to significantly lessen the impact of cerebral palsy and other degenerative diseases. It was also recommended that additional research be done to investigate whether improved modification was possible if the physical therapy regime was increased to multiple times per week on high-risk infants.

Mayo's (1991) initial conclusions have been shown as highly insightful, as recent research in pediatric physical therapy indicates that the detrimental effects of cerebral palsy in infants can be significantly reduced when participation in physical therapy is increased. Damiano (2006) indicates that soft tissue and the central nervous system can be remodeled through participation in physical therapy. Moreover, Damiano (2006) believed that these benefits were not just applicable to infants and young children but could be observed in adults with fully-developed cerebral palsy. The information presented in the research study suggests that physical therapy, strength training, and general activity showed beneficial outcomes for persons with cerebral palsy.

Finally, the evidence supports the use of physical therapy as a strategy to promote improved physiological status through remodeling the physical stature of the individual. Cameron, Maehle, and Reid (2005) explored the outcomes of physical therapy on infants who had been born as "very preterm, very low birth weight" (p. 107). A physical therapy intervention was applied in which the infants in an experimental group received exposure to physical therapy. After four months, the researchers compared the motor performance to that of infants in a control group and found that infants in the experimental group exhibited no abnormal motor development, while 16% of the infants in the control group had demonstrated abnormal motor development. Also, the researchers noted that the infants in the physical therapy group had increased soft tissue mass. The researchers recommended that follow-up research to compare the effects of physical therapy on both groups needed to be carried out to fully understand the impact that physical therapy had on influencing the development of normal motor performance and soft tissue mass.

Physical Fitness and Soft Tissue Healing

The composition of soft tissue differs according to the type of muscle fiber and the physical fitness of the person. Physical conditioning plays a significant role in the rate of recovery (Glaer & Hosey, 2004). Athletes who have conditioned their bodies tend to have soft tissue with greater lean muscle mass than persons who have not engaged in physical conditioning. Persons who are overweight or are obese typically have more fatty deposits in their soft tissues, which can affect the rate of recovery. Goodell (2000) notes that overweight patients, especially those who are obese or morbidly obese, tend to create special challenges for medical care professionals. According to Glaer & Hosey (2004);

Adaptations in hygiene, pharmacologic management, pulmonary support, rehabilitation, prevention of complications, and injury detection are needed to provide effective care to injured obese people. Body habits, technical limitations of equipment, and unique injury patterns may increase the risk of missed injuries in this population. (p. 13)

It is widely accepted that the obese patient is more likely to pose challenges to medical health professionals (Goodell, 2000; Iezzoni, McCarthy, Davis, & Siebens, 2001; Glazer & Hosey, 2004). These patients are at risk for developing soft tissue injury in general and delayed muscle onset soreness in particular because their weight places an additional physical burden on their bodies. Mobility is restricted and the patients are at risk for injuries of the lower extremities because of weight-associated stress centered on these regions (Iezzoni et al., 2001; Glazer & Hosey, 2004). When the obese patient's weight exceeds his or her physical tolerance, mobility difficulties, such as stress factors or soft tissue injury, can result (Iezzoni et al., 2001).

Physical therapists frequently encounter delayed onset muscle soreness from obese persons who have taken steps to improve their physical fitness. Obese patients who begin exercising often do so without recognizing that their bodies have not been prepared to accept changes in lifestyle habits. The obese person who begins to engage in rigorous physical activity without taking the time to gradually prepare his or her body for exercise is prone to injury (Goodell, 2000; Iezzoni et al., 2001; Glazer & Hosey, 2004). Physical therapists who work with obese patients note that their patients are resistant to therapy and attribute the damage they have received to their brief exposure to physical exercise (Dreeben, 2006). It is likely that physical therapists who work with obese patients will have to spend additional time motivating the patient to complete therapeutic exercise, as the patient might demonstrate opposition and unwillingness to alter his or her behavioral habits.

Conversely, obese patients who participate in physical therapy receive multiple benefits. Not only does physical therapy help target injury and improve mobility, but it can help obese patients become familiar with physical exercise. Obese and morbidly obese patients who follow a physical fitness regime learn how to manage their physical fitness through setting aside time for exercise. They can improve their physical fitness through participating in low impact physical therapy exercises and learning techniques that will reduce their risk for future injury. At the conclusion of therapy, obese patients who dedicated themselves to their exercises might demonstrate improved physical fitness and will be better able to manage their own health care regimes.

In contrast to obese persons, athletes have been shown to have a more positive response to physical therapy (Jewell, 2007). Evidence-based practice in physical therapy demonstrates that athletes are more responsive to physical therapy, are more likely to continue the required exercises without oversight, and are more likely to use appropriate independent healing strategies such as applying heat or maintaining rigidity, as recommended by their physicians and therapists (Jewell, 2007). There is also evidence to suggest that soft tissue, which has better overall composition and consistency, is able to heal more rapidly than soft tissue that contains fatty deposits or other characteristics associated with soft tissue that has not been exposed to exercise.

As noted, the type of soft tissue injury can influence the healing process. For example, soft tissue infections require different care and management strategies than damage caused through overextension or compression (Stevens, et al., 2005). All soft tissue injuries can require specialization of therapy, but some types of soft tissue injury appear to be more responsive to therapy than others. Stanish (1984) initially noted that overuse injuries in athletes did not respond well to traditional treatment strategies that are used to manage soft tissue injury in patients who are not athletic. Specifically, Stanish (1984) found that "forced rest or immobilization result in predictable musculoskeletal atrophy with impaired function" and recommended that the soft tissue of athletes responded favorably to treatment strategies that improved mobilization and functionality (p. 1).

Overuse injuries in athletes are a subject of interest to researchers and medical care professionals who study soft tissue injuries that occur from routine activities. As opposed to acute soft tissue injuries caused by non-routine misuse or overextension of the body, routine overuse injuries are the result of normal activities performed by the athlete during training or competition. Overuse injuries are typically associated with structural injuries, and soft tissue damage through overuse is most frequently observed in the joints. However, some muscular overuse injuries are observed, such as damage to the soft tissue of the back and spine. It has also been observed that overuse injuries are the result of "exposure to a high training load [including] duration, frequency, or...distance" (Yeung & Yeung, 2001, p. 383). When injury occurs as the result of soft tissue overuse, some sort of intervention strategy is required to ensure that the injury does not return. These interventions typically involve changing the athlete's training schedule to reduce the chance of overuse (Yeung &

Yeung, 2001). In some instances, physical therapy has been applied to reduce pain and to rebuild the soft tissue to reduce the likelihood of overuse (Glaer & Hosey, 2004; Stevens et al., 2005).

Finally, the patient's age can influence the rate of healing. Overuse soft tissue injuries that have been observed in children appear to heal more quickly than similar injuries that are observed in adults (DiFiori, 1999). Reliance on rapid healing does not, however, mean that children and adolescents aren't at risk for developing chronic damage as the result of soft tissue injury. Pediatric sports injuries can have serious consequences for the developing child's physical status (DiFiori, 1999). Conversely, elderly persons who receive soft tissue injuries are less likely to heal as quickly and are less receptive to physical therapy (Jewell, 2007). Here, the receptiveness of the patient refers not only to the patient's physical health and healing response but the willingness of the patient to engage in self-directed therapeutic exercises (Jewell, 2007).

Specialization of Soft Tissue Sites and Injury Treatment

While the physical fitness of the patient plays a role in recovery and responsiveness to physical therapy, the type of soft tissue that has been damaged by injury can affect the healing process (Makofsky, 2003). Through extensive trial and error, physical therapists have refined their techniques and have developed specialized therapies that target soft tissue injury at specific sites. Spinal manual therapy, for example, has been developed to address soft tissue injury surrounding the spine. Makofsky (2003) notes that the physiological motion of the spine requires substantial support from the surrounding soft tissue, as:

Each of the 24 vertebrae (7 cervical, 12 thoracic, and 5 lumbar) have the ability to move in four places of reference. These motions include forward bending or flexion, backward bending or extension, side bending or lateral flexation to the right and left, and rotation to the right and left (p. 2).

The range of motion required by the spine, especially when coupled with the need to support this motion using multiple muscle groups, makes the spine especially vulnerable to soft tissue injury (Makofsky, 2003). In addition to increased vulnerability, soft tissue damage to the spinal area has historically proven to be chronic injury, as recovery from injury might be limited or the patient is prone to re-injury at the site. It is not fully known how, why, or to what extent soft tissue in the spinal area is less vulnerable to healing than other muscle groups, although health care professionals believe that the extensive soft tissue mass that supports the spine and the constant demands on the spinal region make it difficult to promote a full, permanent cure for soft tissue damage in this region (Makofsky, 2003).

To compensate for the repeating tendencies of re-injury of soft tissue injury at the spine, physical therapists have developed exercises that promote the rule of superior motion (Makofsky, 2003). Segmented motion at the spine stems from the vertebrae, meaning that the rule of superior motion is focused on promoting healing at the spine radiating outward. While damage to soft tissue might extend to different sites throughout the lower torso, upper torso, and neck, all physical therapy targeting these soft tissue groups begins at the spine and radiates outward. The rationale that governs the rule of superior motion is that the spine is included in all physiological functioning involving the soft tissue of the torso, and targeting the spine will thus target the soft tissue injury, even if the injury is not directly connected to soft tissue supported by the vertebrae. By educating the patient in exercises that follow the rule of superior motion, the physical therapist helps the patient recondition all soft tissue associated with the spine and the reconditioning process helps reduce the likelihood of re-injury at both the site of the original damage and in other soft tissue sites that are associated with the spine.

Specialization of therapy has also been applied to diseases or disorders in which soft tissue injury is sustained. For instance, Damiano (2006) argued that physical therapy was of benefit for patients suffering from cerebral palsy. Physical therapy has long been a component of the treatment regimens for patients with cerebral palsy, as it is used to maintain mobility and reduce pain associated with motion. However, Damiano (2006) suggests that specialization of specific physical therapy regimes could be used to improve the patient's overall physical activity. In respect to patients with cerebral palsy, there needs to be a "more focused and proactive approach of promoting activity through more intense active training protocols, lifestyle modifications, and mobility-enhancing devices" (p. 1534). If these changes are made to the traditional physical therapy regime, Damiano (2006) believes that it is possible to affect changes in the quality-of-life of the cerebral palsy patient and improve the patient's overall physical fitness.

Physical Therapy Supplemented with Pharmacological Therapy

The use of pharmacological substances in physical therapy is not limited to pain management. Physical therapy is frequently supplemented with compounds, such as muscle relaxants or steroids to influence the regeneration of the soft tissue. The effectiveness of physical therapy can be improved through supplemental pharmacological therapy, and therapists and physicians work together to find a treatment regime that improves the patient's time in recovery.

The uses for these supplemental compounds are myriad and are determined by the patient's case history and the health care practitioner's knowledge of effective supplemental pharmacological therapy in similar cases. Soft tissue injury accompanied by the risk of infection is the single greatest soft tissue injury requiring supplemental medication, as it is necessary to boost the patient's immune system and reduce the risk of infection through the use of anti-infection medications (Andreasen, Green, & Childers, 2001).

The use of supplements has, however, been questioned by some researchers. Many supplements have benefits for the patients and improve certain aspects of the healing process but have a profound negative impact on other areas of healing. For instance, Dahners and Mullis (2004) explored whether nonsteroidal anti-inflammatory drugs should be administered to patients with both soft-tissue damage and injury to bones. The researchers perceived that while these drugs were beneficial for patients with soft tissue damage, the drugs "diminish bone formation, healing, and remodeling" (p. 139). Patients who were prescribed nonsteroidal anti-inflammatory drugs were therefore put at risk for developing worsening bone damage over time, even though the drugs themselves promoted soft tissue growth. The researchers found that "some nonsteroidal anti-inflammatory drugs have a positive effect on soft-tissue healing; they stimulate collagen synthesis and can increase strength in the early phases of repair during skin and ligament healing" (Dahners and Mullis, 2004, p. 139). Yet while these drugs promoted soft tissue healing, they reduced fracture healing and spine fusion and "may have an adverse effect of ligament healing" (Dahners and Mullis, 2004, p. 139).

Physical Therapy and its Effect on Delayed Onset Muscle Soreness

Physical therapy in the treatment of delayed onset muscle soreness is used to address the inflammation and irritability of damaged tissue. The most common uses of physical therapy in managing inflammation and irritability occur after the patient has suffered physical injury that resulted in acute damage to soft tissue, such as what occurs after a car accident or from chronic conditions, such as repeating lower back pain. Physical therapy is used to help patients learn how to strengthen the existing soft tissue, to help rejuvenate the soft tissue at the site of the damage, and to teach the patient how to move in ways that reduce the risk of re-injuring the site (Kisner & Colby, 2007). Evidence in research studies suggests that physical therapy can have a positive outcome on soft tissue modification, especially when administered to infants and young children.

Resistance Exercise

Physical therapy has been used to treat muscle soreness through the use of resistance exercise. These resistance exercises are determined by negative resistance or positive resistance, which refers to the type of motion used by the muscles as they follow a specific range of motion. Progressive resistance exercise (PRE) incorporates both positive and negative resistance in a preset range of exercises (Taylor, Dodd, & Damiano, 2005). Progressive resistance exercise contains three basic principles, which are (1) to perform a small number of repetitions until fatigue, (2) to allow sufficient rest between exercises for recovery, and (3) to increase the resistance as the ability to generate force increases (Taylor et al., 2006, p. 209). Exercise and therapy that use these principles of PRE are formally applied to increase strength, although informal applications of PRE are found throughout general and specialized physical therapy regimes, as "between 52% and 69% of physical therapy treatments for spinal impairment included 'strengthening' exercises and that up to 87% of treatments for knee impairments included 'strengthening' exercises" (Taylor et al., 2006, p. 209). It has been argued that PRE is a necessary part of physical therapy, as improving the capacity of the muscles to react to environmental stimuli is believed to reduce the stress placed on the soft tissue when reactions are required (Makofsky, 2003). However, PRE has been widely criticized as being misused in physical therapy as "there have been concerns that training muscles to increase force production could have a negative effect by increasing muscle spasticity" and that "in musculoskeletal physical therapy, safety concerns have been raised about the application of relatively high forces requiring PRE training through healing tissues, such as through bone after fracture" (Taylor et al., 2006, p. 209).

In respect to muscle soreness, PRE has been used to improve the capacity of soft tissue to withstand stress (Makofsky, 2003; Kinser & Colby, 2006; Taylor et al., 2006). When incorporated into physical therapy, it is believed that PRE serves as a preventative therapy as it helps improve the fitness and the lean muscle mass of soft tissue. If this is true, then progressive resistance exercise thus enhances the composition of soft tissue and increases its resiliency (Kinser & Coby, 2006). Unfortunately, PRE does not yield these benefits over the short term and must be used consistently and with progressive increases in resistance to yield beneficial results (Kinser & Coby, 2006).

Research has also shown that PRE can be used to rehabilitate persons who suffered from neurological impairments. Ouellette, et al. (2004) found that persons who had suffered a stroke demonstrated improved muscular control after participating in PRE. The researchers noted that improved control was mainly observed in increased strength and improved motor control in small tasks but that "the present study found no chances in functional performance despite improvements in strength and power" (p. 1408). The outcome was one in which physical therapy did appear to assist the affected person in regaining neuromuscular control, but there were limits on the benefits.

Balance Training

Impaired balance is associated with reduced healing time for soft tissue damage. Impaired balance generally does not result in problems for persons suffering from muscle soreness but can cause additional injury as the result of falling or can place stress on other muscles as the patient compensates for limited mobility by engaging in unnatural or non-habitual movements (e.g. limping, slouching, etc.). Balance training in physical therapy can help persons who have suffered from soft tissue injury learn how to maintain mobility without placing them at risk for exacerbating the original injury (Kinser & Coby, 2006). The majority of the research in balance training is done on the elderly, as balance training is used to purposefully reduce the risk of falls among elderly persons. However, balance training has also been used for younger persons and athletes to improve the neuromuscular control of the body. Holme, et al. (1998) found that balance training was highly effective in preventing re-injury among athletes who had experienced acute ankle ligament sprain. The researchers believed that re-injury typically affected those athletes who attempted to reduce pain through overcompensating for their injuries in different muscle groups. Doing so merely reduced the likelihood that the injured soft tissue would receive effective rehabilitation and would promote re-injury once the affected soft tissue was used.

Pain Management for Patients with Delayed Onset Muscle Soreness

Acute muscle soreness occurs as the result of overuse or overextension of soft tissue (Kinser & Coby, 2006). Delayed muscle onset soreness occurs as a result of acute damage to soft tissue, but the repairs to the injury are typically associated with pain through tissue regeneration or because of secondary causes such as inflammation or irritation (Kinser & Coby, 2006). As patients often seek out physical therapy because they experience pain, the physical therapist is aware that such patients want to reduce or eliminate their pain through physical therapy. The physical therapist works closely with the patient's physician to help identify appropriate pain management strategies, including the management of inflammation and irritation, as well as pain resulting from infection and secondary soft tissue damage.

There is substantial research to suggest that physical therapy is beneficial in reducing symptoms of pain in patients with soft tissue injury, but these benefits are experienced over time. To restate, Herring's (1990) five goals of the physical therapy process include; (1) establishment of an accurate diagnosis, (2) minimization of deleterious local effects of the acute injury, (3) allowance for proper healing, (4) maintenance of other components of athletic fitness, and (5) return to normal athletic function (p. 453). These are not immediate outcomes and require time and effort on the part of the patient, the patient's primary care physician, and the patient's physical therapist. Research has shown that pain management is improved for patients who incorporate physical therapy into their healing regimes, but the outcomes are not immediately apparent (Sinclair, Hogg-Johnson, Mondloch, & Shields, 1997). Physical therapy has thus not been used to treat pain associated with acute muscle soreness or delayed onset muscle soreness. This section explores alternative strategies that have been put into use to help patients manage pain associated with delayed onset muscle soreness.

Inflammation and Irritation in Pain Management

Inflammation and irritation are the single greatest causes of pain for patients suffering from delayed onset muscle soreness (Kisner & Colby, 2006). Patients suffering from chronic injury have persistent inflammation and irritation, while patients who have acute injury are more likely to suffer mainly from inflammation with some minor irritation (Kisner & Colby, 2006). Arthritis is the single most common form of chronic soft tissue injury that requires pain management (Dieppe & Lohmander, 2005). The second most common form of soft tissue injury that requires pain management is caused by infection (Bisno & Stevens, 1996).

Athletes who experience soft tissue injury are more likely to experience different types of inflammation and irritation than non-athletes (d'Hemecourt, Gerbino, & Micheli, 2000). The athlete is more likely to experience muscle soreness than a non-athlete, as well as pain in soft tissues such as tendons, joints, ligaments, and other soft tissues that are involved in physical activities (d'Hemecourt et al., 2000; Yeung & Yeung, 2001). Delayed onset muscle soreness is a common source of pain among athletes. Cleak and Eston (1992) postulated a similar argument to that of d'Hemecourt et al. (2000), noting that athletes who have undergone extensive physical conditioning are more likely to experience muscle contractions that exacerbate pain in the soft tissue. Simply, the mechanisms of conditioned muscles have increased the mass of the soft tissue, and corresponding exposure to physical activity ensures that athletes use the muscles more often than non-athletes. Thus, athletes are more likely to be exposed to conditions that could cause or contribute to delayed onset muscle soreness and have greater soft tissue mass that can sustain injury.

Pain management of delayed onset muscle soreness often incorporates steroidal treatments to reduce swelling and inflammation. However, many athletes are resistant to the use of steroids in their training regimes, as the use of some steroidal compounds is viewed by sporting associations as a violation of performance standards. Athletes are more likely to use non-steroidal anti-inflammatory drugs to reduce swelling and inflammation; while these are not as effective as steroidal compounds, they do not have an associated risk of punishment for violating performance standards. Lippi, Franchini, and Guidi (2006) indicated that there are other risks associated with non-steroidal pain management, such as increased risk of internal bleeding. Aspirin, a compound that is commonly used to treat pain is an example of a pharmacological substance that increases the patient's risk of bleeding but is frequently used to treat delayed onset muscle soreness by reducing inflammation (Lippi et al., 2006).

Cheung, Hume, and Maxwell (2003) note that the most effective strategy for reducing delayed onset muscle soreness in athletes is through effective planning and preparation. Most incidences of delayed onset muscle soreness in athletes are the result of athletes following poorly-planned exercise routines or failing to prepare for new athletic seasons and other activities. The researchers find that delayed onset muscle soreness is "most prevalent at the beginning of the sporting season when athletes are returning to training following a period of reduced activity" and it is "also common when athletes are first introduced to certain types of activities regardless of the time of year" (Cheung, Hume, and Maxwell, 2003, p. 45). The researchers suggested that the "micro-injuries" to the muscle can be alleviated if the athlete is physically prepared to engage in physical activity. However, Cheung et al (2003) also noted that treatment strategies that are widely accepted as beneficial in healing soft tissue injuries have not been effective in either reducing pain or promoting healing, where "cryotherapy, stretching, homeopathy, ultrasound, and electrical current modalities have demonstrated no effect on the alleviation of muscle soreness or other delayed onset muscle soreness symptoms" (p. 145). The most effective strategy that reduces pain caused by delayed onset muscle soreness is exercise, but "the analgesic effect is also temporary" and it is possible that increased exercise can exacerbate existing injury (Cheung et al., 2003, p. 145). Subsequently, the treatment that is most often used for reducing pain in delayed onset muscle soreness is to reduce exercise but not eliminate it altogether (Ernst, 1998; Cheung et al., 2003).

Alternative Techniques for Pain Management with Delayed Onset Muscle Soreness

Physical therapists working with patients prone to suffering delayed onset muscle soreness recognize that patients require therapeutic intervention to reduce pain and to promote healing in soft tissue sites. As delayed onset, muscle soreness is almost always a response to acute injury, efforts to promote pain management incorporate the knowledge that the soft tissue injury is temporary, and that healing the injury is the best strategy for pain management (Weber, Servedio, & Woodall, 1994). However, some alternative therapies have been proposed that might help alleviate the pain associated with delayed onset muscle soreness. There is evidence that therapeutic massage can be used to help reduce pain. Ernst (1998) explored how post-exercise massage cold be applied to facilitate pain management for subjects who had engaged in activities that were likely to induce delayed onset muscle soreness. Ernst drew upon a large body of literature in which the effects of massage therapy had been studied on athletes. The research by Ernst had serious inconsistencies in methodology but did suggest that massage applied directly to the affected soft tissue immediately following exercise was likely to reduce pain and stiffness associated with delayed onset muscle soreness. Ernst theorized that massaging soft tissue would restrict the effects of delayed onset muscle soreness because massage interfered with the pathophysiology of the condition. The researcher outlined the six commonly held hypotheses used to explain the pathophysiology associated with delayed onset muscle soreness:

(1) Exercise leads to local accumulation of metabolic waste, which in turn sensitizes A-delta and C fibers causing pain.

(2) Exercise causes muscle ischaemia, which results in the production of a pain substance. Pain in turn produces a reflex spasm which, in a vicious cycle, prolongs ischaemia.

(3) Exercise results in intramuscular edema, which activates mechanoreceptors thus causing pain.

(4) Eccentric exercise leads to damage of the connective tissues in the area of the muscle and this damage is responsible for the pain.

(5) Exercise leads to the release of inflammatory byproducts, which sensitizes nerve fibers thus causing pain.

(6) Exercise leads to destruction within muscle fibers liberating muscle creatine kinase, which is the cause of pain (pp. 213-214).

Ernst (1998) postulated that massage could interfere with all six of these processes, where "through its mechanical pressure on muscle tissue, massage treatment leads to enhanced local microcirculatory blood and lymph flow. This, in turn, reduces edema, ischaemia, or accumulation of substances that directly or indirectly causes pain" (p. 214). Additional research into massage therapy was needed to explore not only how massage affected the symptoms of delayed onset muscle soreness but also how it affected physiological processes associated with pain.

Five years later, Farr, Nottle, Nosaka, and Sacco (2002) conducted the type of study recommended by Ernst (1998). Farr et al. (2002) found that therapeutic massage is beneficial in alleviating pain by inducing conditions favorable for delayed onset muscle soreness and applying therapeutic massage. Eight male subjects volunteered to use a treadmill for 40 minutes and carrying equipment that comprised "ten percent of their body mass" (p. 297). Following the exercise regime, "a qualified masseur performed a 30-min therapeutic massage to one limb tow hours post-walk" (p. 279). The researchers assessed the patients for "muscle soreness, tenderness, isometric strength, isokinetic strength, and single leg vertical jump height" and measured these "before, and 1, 24, 72 and 120-hours post-walk for both limbs" (p. 297). The researchers found that there were significant differences in reports of pain experienced by the subjects in the leg that had received the therapeutic massage and concluded that therapeutic massage immediately after muscle exertion would reduce the impact of delayed onset muscle soreness.

Summary

Physical therapy has an impact on soft tissue healing. It has traditionally been applied after an acute injury has had time to begin the healing process and is used to promote the health and recovery of soft tissue. There are many different forms of soft tissue healing and physical therapy strategies have been adapted for specialized treatment of certain forms of soft tissue damage. The physical composition of the soft tissue can affect the rate of healing and the patient's relationship to physical therapy, especially when the patient is athletic or obese or has a disorder that affects the soft tissue, such as cerebral palsy. There is some evidence to suggest that massage therapies can reduce conditions associated with delayed onset muscle soreness. Pharmacological therapy and physical therapy have been shown to reduce pain by reducing inflammation and the risk of infection. Exercise and increased mobility have been found to provide the most effective relief from pain caused by delayed onset muscle soreness, even though this relief is temporary. However, the causes of delayed onset muscle soreness are not fully understood and it is not known whether physical therapy can be used immediately following acute injury to assist in pain management.

CHAPTER V:
SUMMARY, DISCUSSION, RECOMMENDATION, AND CONCLUSION

Physical therapy is applied for patients who suffer from somatic dysfunction, which is the impairment of the musculo-skeletal system. However, while physical therapy is centered in medical practice and governed by medical research, there is an undeniable human-centered component to physical therapy. In 1987, Leon Chaitow noted in the classic handbook for physical therapists, *Soft Tissue Manipulation*, that there is a "subjective value" to all physical therapy (p. 1). The practitioner, Chaitow (1987), noted does not touch a patient and recognize the presence of conditions that are described in the medical literature as stringy, nodular, or indurated (p. 1). Chaitow (1987) believed that while patient care can be guided by the research and the physical therapist's education but in large part is governed almost exclusively by the patient's unique case history and the physical therapist's professional experience.

The current research paper has sought to explore whether soft tissue damage, specifically soft tissue damage as the result of delayed onset muscle soreness following exercise can be managed through physical therapy. As soft tissue damage is a somatic dysfunction, physical therapy is frequently used in treating the injury after it has occurred. It is widely accepted that patients who receive physical therapy for soft tissue injury demonstrate more comprehensive recovery from soft tissue damage and recovery is attained more quickly than if physical therapy was not used. However, physical therapy is typically used to help manage the recovery process and is not applied as a part of the treatment regime immediately following the injury. While physical therapy is used to help improve the rehabilitation and fitness of soft tissue after injury, it is not yet known whether physical therapy can be used immediately after injury as an initial treatment to reduce pain and to promote healing.

This final chapter presents the results of the information discovered through the use of a grounded literature review methodology used to assess the literature on soft tissue healing through the application of physical therapy. A summary of the main topics in the paper is used to introduce the chapter and a discussion of the findings used to address the utility of physical therapy in treating soft tissue damage. The conclusion will provide an assessment of the findings, recommendations for application, and areas of inquiry that have to be considered in future research studies.

Summary

The research project sought to explore the applications of physical therapy as a means of promoting healing among patients who suffered soft tissue injury with accompanying delayed onset muscle soreness. The problem statement that governed the research process was:

> Healing regimes traditionally incorporate physical therapy after an initial recovery period has reduced the traumatic effects associated with impairment or injury, but the careful and appropriate introduction of physical therapy at an earlier period in a healing regime may potentially speed up the initial healing process.

A grounded literature review was used to collect data that clarified the role of soft tissue injury, pain management, and the healing process in the context of physical therapy. Three research questions were used to guide the data collection process:

1. What is the role of physical therapy in soft tissue healing?
2. What is the impact of physical therapy on delayed onset muscle soreness?

3. Does instruction in physical therapy help persons suffering from delayed onset muscle soreness manage their pain?

It has been found that delayed onset muscle soreness has proven challenging for physical therapists who strive to provide treatment regimens that help patients manage pain and improve physical fitness (Weber et al., 1994). Delayed onset muscle soreness is typically the result of inflammation of the muscles but can also be caused by infection or secondary injuries such as overextension (Kisner & Colby, 2007). Pain management of delayed onset muscle soreness is typically managed through pain medications that target the reflex actions that cause pain and pain management achieved not through treating the injury itself but through reducing the severity of symptoms such as inflammation or infection. Physicians' attitudes toward pain management differ according to the patient's unique case history and the physician's training and experience in pain management for similar cases. Patients who suffer from diseases or disorders that are typically associated with pain, such as cancer or acute injury due to severe trauma, are more likely to receive therapeutic pain management using pharmaceuticals. Patients who are more susceptible to pain, such as children and the elderly, are also more likely to receive pain management therapy using medications than patients who are younger or who are in better overall physical shape. Similarly, patients have differing attitudes towards pain based upon their physiological response to symptoms of pain, their opinions of how they should manage their personal quality-of-life, and other personal attitudes towards pain and the perception of pain.

Pain management through pharmaceuticals is not used to treat the pain but affects the patient's perception of pain. Patients who receive pain management medication are managing their pain through reducing their awareness of acute activation of sensory information. However, pain management is recognized as a highly ambiguous process and the sensations of pain differ on a case-to-case basis. Health care professionals involved in pain management recognize that the assessment of pain and the management of pain symptoms cannot be generalized and that patients' responses to pain differ throughout the course of their disease or injury.

Physical therapists are typically not licensed physicians and cannot prescribe prescription drugs for pain medication, which limits their control of patients' pain management. The therapist works closely with the patient's physician and can make recommendations for pain management based upon the patient's case history and progress made during therapy. Unfortunately, there appear to be deficits in therapists' understanding of pain management and perceptions of how pain should best be addressed among patients, suggesting that therapists might require additional education and training in pain management therapy.

Pain management is of concern to physicians, patients, and other health care professionals because effective pain management through the use of pharmaceuticals has been closely associated with addiction. The most effective pain management medications are accompanied by the risk of addiction because the effects of such substances on the brain not only characterizes the patient's perception of pain but is also associated with hormonal responses that provide physiological rewards for the patient. As the risk of addiction to pain management medications increases when the patient suffers from high levels from pain or is not in a position where he or she can manage access to medication (e.g. in intensive care in a hospital), some patients are at greater risk of developing addiction than others.

Management of pain associated with soft tissue injury is a complex process. Soft tissue injury can be acute or chronic and can be caused through exposure to external stimuli or through internal actions that stress the soft tissue beyond its existing limitations on mobility. Pain associated with soft tissue injury differs according to the nature of the injury, but pain caused by both acute and chronic soft tissue injury can be severe. Treatment for all acute soft tissue injury includes protection, rest, ice, compression, elevation, and support, while chronic injury in the soft tissue can be managed through these and other therapies, such as cryotherapy. As all soft tissue injury is at risk of exacerbation due to inflammation and infection, the treatment used depends on the nature of the injury. Surgery can be used to manage pain, especially if the soft tissue has suffered extensive damage and requires restructuring or removal to reduce the damage and promote healing.

Physical therapy could potentially be used as a means of promoting healing among patients who suffer acute soft tissue injuries. Manipulation and mobilization of the site of soft tissue damage has been shown to be beneficial for persons suffering from certain forms of soft tissue injury. Massage has also been found to help improve mobility and reduce pain and does not tend to exacerbate the injury. Physical therapy incorporates principles of manipulation, mobilization, and massage, in addition to improving muscle fitness and strength. However, the nature of the injury might create special considerations for the physical therapist and for the patient alike; healing might be affected by the patient's physical condition, the location of the injury, and the type of soft tissue affected and additional strategies used to supplement the healing process such as pharmacological therapy. However, there are potential negative outcomes that accompany the use of pharmacological therapy, such as non-steroidal anti-inflammatory drugs damaging soft tissue.

While most methods of physical therapy are appropriate for treating soft tissue damage, there is dispute over which forms of physical therapy yield the best outcomes. Resistance therapy can have beneficial results for some forms of soft tissue damage, but it can also exacerbate the site of the existing injury. Some researchers support the use of physical therapy to promote healing, but there remain questions regarding whether immediate healing can occur. Researchers who tested the rate of healing in persons who were affected by muscle damage have found that there is no observable difference between subjects who receive physical therapy and those who do not. Sinclair, Hogg-Johnson, Mondloch, and Shields (1997) tested the relationship between patients with soft tissue injury who received physical therapy immediately after injury. The research showed that patients who participated in an experimental physical therapy program were no more likely to demonstrate appropriate healing than patients who did not.

Discussion

The current research study has sought to test whether pain as caused by delayed onset muscle soreness could be managed through treating the injury as opposed to the symptoms. Traditional pain management targets the symptoms of injury, especially inflammation, infection, and secondary stress that exacerbate the original injury. If physical therapy can be used to promote healing of the original injury without causing additional harm to the patient, then it is possible that physical therapy could be applied as an alternative to medication as used in traditional pain management strategies.

The research process has shown that the literature on physical therapy as a means of treating acute injury is sadly lacking. Information on acute injury and the subsequent pain expressed by such injuries does not reveal the effectiveness of physical therapy as appropriate as an immediate response to injury. With that said, there is evidence to support the use of physical therapy as a healing technique (Houghlum, 1992). Cheung et al., (2003) stressed that if pain medications will not be used, then exercise and movement are the most effective strategies to reduce pain caused by delayed onset muscle soreness. The evidence also indicates that restricted physical activity following delayed onset muscle soreness will help keep soft tissues from becoming immobile and rigid (Weber et al., 1994; Cheung et al., 2003; Taylor et al., 2006). Soft tissue massage has shown positive results in respect to healing soft tissue damage (Ernst, 1998; Mikesky & Hayden, 2005). While acute injury is not covered in the research, these traits all serve to indicate that physical therapy can be used to reduce pain, promote flexibility, and improve healing, which can be components of successful management of acute injury.

The review of the literature suggests that there is a clear need to investigate the application of physical therapy as a catalyst in soft tissue healing or as an agent that promotes healing and alleviates pain. Cheung et al., (2003) noted that while the mechanisms of soft tissue injury have been thoroughly documented and the causes of delayed onset muscle soreness are recognized, there is very little evidence to guide acute care. There is a need for strategies that reduce pain and promote healing as traditional strategies, such as cryotherapy, and more recent strategies, such as ultrasound, are not effective (Cheung et al., 2003). If it is shown that physical therapy can be used as an effective strategy to promote healing and alleviate pain, then there is incentive to apply physical therapy for patients with delayed onset muscle soreness.

Unfortunately, physical therapy, as it is currently used in the health care setting, is structured for use after the acute injury has passed and the soft tissue has had time to recover from trauma (Jette, 1995; Almekinders, 1996; Haetzman et al., 2003; Kisner & Coby, 2006). As there are multiple forms of physical therapy, it is plausible that a new type of physical therapy can be adapted and applied to acute injury. Physical therapy has the ability to improve healing by educating the patient in appropriate methods of movement (Chaitow, 1987). Adapted applications of physical therapy were observed in the applications of massage after physical exertion, where the pain of delayed onset muscle soreness was reduced and recovery from injury was more rapid (Ernst, 1998; Farr et al., 2003; Nadler, 2004). These outcomes suggest that it is plausible that physical therapy can be used to treat acute soft tissue injury and make it probable that physical therapy can be applied to manage the pain associated with delayed onset muscle soreness. These likelihoods aside, the lack of evidence in the use of physical therapy exclusively as a treatment for acute soft tissue injury prevents the researcher from concluding that physical therapy is appropriate in this context. Additional research is required before physical therapy is shown to be appropriate to promote healing and reduce pain in delayed onset muscle soreness.

Recommendations

The results of the grounded literature review show that more research is needed before it can be concluded that physical therapy is an appropriate healing and pain management fitness regime for managing delayed onset muscle soreness immediately after exertion occurs. There is very little evidence that specifically targets the use of physical therapy as a cure for immediate acute pain. However, there is an abundance of information that clearly shows that physical therapy is useful both as a strategy to prevent additional injury and as an effective form of long-term pain management. Applying physical therapy to acute soft tissue damage immediately after this damage has occurred might have multiple benefits for the patient, including improved pain management, increased mobility and muscle tone, and reduced likelihood that the patient will overextend or overuse the affected soft tissue.

It is possible that these benefits can be applied to treat delayed onset muscle soreness immediately after the incident has occurred, but it is most likely that the results of application will only be observed in patients who are already familiar with physical therapy techniques. Patients who are aware of how physical therapy functions and routinely practice physical therapy will already possess the skills and education required to implement physical therapy are able to do so immediately after injury; patients who are unaware of physical therapy techniques and have never used them first need to receive instruction in these techniques and then learn how to apply them while suffering from soft tissue injury.

Here, research into whether physical therapy can be used to promote healing of soft tissue damage meets a stumbling block. It is accepted that applying physical therapy can result in pain for the affected patient (Kannus, 2000; Taylor et al., 2006; Kisner & Colby, 2006). Pain occurs from the use of soft tissue or bone that has been injured and might also be affected by secondary symptoms, such as inflammation, infection, or strain. It is possible that subjects in the experimental group might experience increased symptoms of pain due to the rigors of physical therapy. It is also possible that engaging in physical therapy immediately following soft tissue injury might exacerbate the injury rather than helping promote healing. Additional ethical considerations must be considered in developing this type of experiment, as it is thus far unknown precisely how physical therapy as used in this manner might impact the subjects in the experiment. It is possible that subjects might exacerbate their injuries and that instead of promoting the healing process, physical therapy might actually prologue it.

Research designed to test whether soft tissue damage can be improved through physical therapy must therefore incorporate control subjects with no knowledge of physical therapy and an experimental group consisting of subjects who receive instruction in specific physical therapy techniques. However, an additional problem can be realized at this point, as physical therapy tends to be specialized to help a patient manage recovery from a specific injury. Efforts to train subjects in effective physical therapy techniques prior to soft tissue injury will likely be generalized and not localized to a specific site or muscle group. To avoid this limitation, it is recommended that future research be applied to persons who routinely suffer from a specific type of soft tissue injury, such as athletes who experience delayed onset muscle soreness in the legs or the arms. With this in mind, the proposed study must use three populations, all of whom are athletes who participate in the same sport and are likely to suffer from similar types of soft tissue damage (e.g. soccer players who are prone to leg injuries, tennis players who are prone to arm soreness, etc.). The subjects in the experimental group can then be instructed in physical therapy techniques that target these areas. The first is a control group that has not learned any physical therapy, the second is an experimental group that has been instructed in physical therapy and who use physical therapy on a routine basis, and the third is an experimental group that have been instructed in physical therapy techniques but have also been instructed to not use these techniques until immediately after injury has occurred. Results of this study will then compare the rate of healing as evidenced by the participants in the three groups. Comparison of the self-reported rate of healing by the subjects will help demonstrate the effect that physical therapy has had on the sample population. All subjects will also report the degree of pain that they experience because of the injury, and those subjects in the experimental groups will report on the nature and the severity of pain they experience prior to, during, and following the application of physical therapy techniques. Then, the results can be used to show how physical therapy influences the rate of healing and recovery for patients suffering soft tissue injury.

Conclusion

Pain management in delayed onset muscle soreness is best achieved through promoting healing at the injury site (Weber et al., 1994). Traditional methods of pain management for delayed onset muscle soreness include reducing inflammation and irritation, which are the primary causes of pain. Physical therapy can also improve mobility and balance, which reduces the likelihood that routine movement, will exacerbate the original injury and prevent secondary injury due to falls or overcompensation by uninjured soft tissue groups. Yet the research study has not demonstrated whether physical therapy will have a positive effect on the causes of pain as associated with delayed onset muscle soreness. There is some evidence that suggests that physical therapy can reduce healing by exacerbating the damage caused to the soft tissue when used immediately after injury. Physical therapy has traditionally been introduced once the patient's injuries have begun to heal, which suggests that the stress induced by physical therapy improves the patient's fitness once recovery has started, and that physical therapy does improve the healing process through improving muscle composition, mobility, flexibility, and educating the patient in how to prevent additional injury. Immediate use of physical therapy following injury might have an adverse effect on the soft tissue at the site of the injury and could restrict the healing process. It is also possible that using physical therapy immediately after injury can result in increased pain for the patient.

With that said, physical therapy continues to be used in new or transformative ways in the health care setting. Physical therapy has been applied to treat soft tissue injury in patients who suffer from both acute and chronic soft tissue damage. Physical therapy is used to manage delayed onset muscle soreness after the pain from the injury has emerged. Patients also routinely report that pain during the physical therapy process is more severe, but following physical therapy, the sensation of pain is reduced. When used to treat certain conditions, such as soft tissue injury of the back, physical therapy also serves to improve muscle tone and muscle composition of the soft tissue both at the site of the injury and in the unaffected soft tissue. These outcomes suggest that there are positive indications that persons prone to specific types of soft tissue injury can receive education and training in physical therapy and develop a physical therapy regime that not only increases their resistance to soft tissue injury but also improves recovery even before the pain of delayed onset muscle soreness makes itself known. It is highly probable that additional research in physical therapy will show its usefulness as a pain prevention strategy, as well as its current application as a rehabilitation tool.

REFERENCES

Abram, S. E. (2004). Test preparation and planning. In M.S. Wallace & P. Staats (Eds.), *Pain Medicine and Management: Just the facts*. New York: McGraw-Hill Professional. (pp. 12-18)

Almekinders, L.C. (1996). *Soft tissue injuries in sports medicine*. New York: Blackwell Science.

Andreasen, T.J., Green, S.D., & Childers, B. (2001). Massive infectious soft-tissue injury: diagnosis and management of necrotizing fasciitis and purpura fulminans. *Plastic and Reconstructive Surgery*, 107(4), 1025-1034.

Aspelin, P., Ejberg, O., Thorsson, O., Wilhelmsson, M., & Westin, N. (1992). Ultrasound examination of soft tissue injury of the lower limb in athletes. *American Journal of Sports Medicine*, 20(5), 601-603.

Bassewitzm H.L. & Shapiro, M.S. (1997). Persistent pain after ankle sprain: targeting the causes. *The Physician and Sports Medicine*, 25(12). Retrieved September 1, 2008, from http://physsportsmed.com/issues/1997/12dec/shapiro.htm

Bender, E. (2007). Painkillers pass pot as drug of choice. *Psychiatric News*, 42, 10.

Bisno, A.L., & Stevens, D.L., (1996). Streptococcal infections of skin and tissues. *New England Journal of Medicine*, 334(4), 240-246.

Bleakley, C., McDonough, S. & MacAuley, D. (2004). The use of ice in the treatment of acute soft-tissue injury: a systematic review of randomized controlled trials. *Scandinavian Journal of Medicine and Science in Sports*, 14(2), 134.

Cameron, E.C, Maehle, V., & Reid, J. (2005). The effects of an early physical therapy intervention for very preterm, very low birth weight infants: a randomized controlled clinical trial. *Pediatric Physical Therapy*, 17(2). 107-119.

Cami, J. & Farre, M. (2003). Drug addition. *New England Journal of Medicine*, 349, 975-986. Chaitow, L. (1987). *Soft tissue manipulation: A practitioner's guide to the diagnosis and treatment of soft-tissue dysfunction and Reflex activity*. New York: Healing Arts Press. Cheung, K., Hume, P.A., & Maxwell, L. (2003). Delayed onset muscle soreness: treatment strategies and performance factors. *Sports Medicine*, 33(2), 145-164.

Cleak, M.J., & Eston, R.G., (1992). Delayed onset muscle soreness: mechanisms and management. *Journal of Sports Science*, 10(4), 325-341.

Dahners, L.E. & Mullis, B.H. (2004). Effects of nonsteroidal anti-inflammatory drugs on bone formation and soft-tissue healing. *American Academy of Orthopedic Surgeons*, 12, 139-143.

Damiano, D.L. (2006). Activity, activity, activity: rethinking our physical therapy approach to cerebral palsy. *Physical Therapy*, 86(11), 1534-1540.

Dieppe, P.A., & Lohmander, L.S., (2005). Pathogenesis and management of pain in osteoarthritis. *Lancet*, 365(9463), 965-973.

DiFidori, J.P. (1999). Overuse injuries in children and adolescents. *Physician and Sports Medicine*, 27(1), 16-21.

Dillin, L., & Slabaugh, P. (1986). Delayed wound healing, infection, and nonunion following open reduction and fixation of tibial plafond fractures. *Journal of Trauma, Injury, Infection, and critical Care*, 26(12), 1116-1119.

Dreeben, O. (2006). *Introduction to physical therapy for physical therapist assistants*, New York: Jones & Bartlett Publishers.

Ernst, E. (1998). Does post-exercise massage treatment reduce delayed onset muscle soreness? A systematic review. *British Journal of Sports Medicine*, 32, 212-214.

Farr, T., Nottle, C., Nosaka, K., & Sacco, P. (2002). The effects of therapeutic massage on delayed onset muscle soreness. *Journal of Science and Medicine in Sport*, 5(4), 297-306. Glaser, B. G. (1998*). Doing grounded theory: Issues and discussions*. New York: Sociology Press.

Glaser, B., & Strauss, A. (1967). *The discovery of grounded theory*. Chicago, IL: Aldine. Glazer, J., & Hosey, R., (2004). Soft tissue injuries of the lower extremity, Primary Care: Clinics in Office Practice, 31(4), 1005-1024.

Goodell, T.T., (2000). The obese trauma patient: treatment strategies. *Australian Emergency Nursing Journal*, 3(2), 13-18.

Gottrup, F, Agren, M.S., & Karlsmark, T. (2000). Models for use in wound healing research: a survey focusing on in vitro and in vivo adult soft tissue. *Wound Repair and Regeneration*, 8(2), 83-96.

Gourlay, D., Heit, H.A., & Almahrezi, A. (2005). Universal precautions in pain medicine: a rational approach to the treatment of chronic pain. *Pain Medicine*, 6(2), 107-112.

Haetzman, M, Elliott, A.M, Smith, B.H., Hannaford, P., & Chambers, W.A., (2003). Chronic pain and the use of conventional and alternative therapy. *Family Practice*, 20(2), 147- 154.

Herring, S.A. (1990). Rehabilitation of muscle injuries. *Medicine & Science in Sports & Exercise*, 22(4), 453-456.

Holme, E., Magnusson, S.P., Becher, K., Bieler, T., Aagaard, P., & Kjaer, M. (1998). The effect of supervised rehabilitation on strength, postural sway, position sense and re-injury risk after acute ankle ligament sprain. *Scandinavian Journal of Medicine and Sciences*, 9(2), 104-109.

Hom, D.B., Thatcher, G., & Tibesar, R. (2002). Growth factor therapy to improve soft tissue healing. *Facial Plastic Surgery*, 18(1), 41-52.

Houglum, P.A. (1992). Soft tissue healing and its impact on rehabilitation. *Journal of Sport Rehabilitation*, 1, 19-39.

Howard, R. F. (2003). Current status of pain management in children. *Journal of the American Medical Association*, 290, 2464-2469.

Hubbard, T.J. & Denegar, C.R. (2004). Does cryotherapy improve outcomes with soft tissue injury? *Journal of Athletic Training*, 39, 274-279.

Iezzoni, L.I., McCarthy, E.P., Davis, R.B., & Siebens, H. (2001). Mobility difficulties are not only a problem of old age. *Journal of General Inter-*

nal Medicine, 16(4), 235-243. Jette, A.M. (1995). Outcomes research: Shifting the dominant research paradigm in physical therapy. *Physical Therapy*, 75(11), 967-970.

Jewell, D.V., (2008). *Guide to evidence-based physical therapy practice*. New York: Jones and Bartlett Publishers, Inc.

Kannus, P. (2000). Immobilization or early mobilization after an acute soft tissue injury? *Physician and Sports Medicine*, 28, 55-63.

Kisner, C., & Colby, L.A., (2006). *Therapeutic exercise: Foundations and techniques* New York: F.S. Davis Company.

Kraemer, W.J., Bush, J.A., Wickham, R.B., Denegar, C.R., Gomez, A.L., Sotshalk, L.A, et al. (2001). Influence of compression therapy on symptoms following soft tissue injury from maximal eccentric exercise. *Journal of Occupational Sports Physical Therapy*, 31(6), 282-290.

Lebovits, A.H., Florence, I., Bathina, R., Hunko, V., Fox, M., & Bramble, C., (1997). Pain knowledge and attitudes of healthcare providers: practice characteristic differences. *Clinical Journal of Pain*, 13(3), 237-243.

Leshner, A. I. (2003). Addition is a brain disease, and it matters. *Focus*, 1, 190–193. Lippi, G., Franchini, M., & Guidi, G.C. (2006). Non-steroidal anti-inflammatory drugs in athletes. *British Journal of Sports Medicine*, 40, 661-663.

Loisel, P., Abenhaim, L., Durand, P., Esdaile, J.M., Suidda, S., Gosselin, L., et.al (1997). A population-based, randomized clinical trial on back pain management. *Spine*. 22(24). 2911-2918.

Makofsky, H.W., (2003). *Spinal manual therapy: An introduction to soft tissue mobilization, spinal manipulation, therapeutic and home exercise*. New York: Slack Incorporated.

Mayo, N. (1991). The effect of physical therapy for children with motor delay and cerebral palsy: A randomized clinical trial. *American Journal of Physical Medicine & Rehabilitation*, 70(5), 116-123.

Mikesky, A., & Hayden, M., (2005). Effect of static management therapy on recovery from delayed onset muscle soreness. *Physical therapy in Sport*, 6(4), 188-194.

Motamedi, M. (2003). Primary management of maxillofacial hard and soft tissue gunshot and shrapnel injuries. *Journal of Oral and Maxillofacial Surgery*, 61(12), 1390-1398. Nadler, S.F. (2004). Nonpharmacological management of pain. *Journal of the American Osteopathic Association*, 104(11), 6-12.

Ouellette, M.M., LeBrasseur, N.K., Bean, J.F., Phillips, E., Stein, J., Frontera, W.R., et.al (2004). High-intensity resistance training improves muscle strength, self-reported function, and disability in long-term stroke survivors. *Stroke*, 35(2), 1404-1409.

Phillips, D.M. (2000). JCAHO pain management standards are unveiled. *Journal of the American Medical Association*, 284, 428-429.

Pinsky, D. (2004). *When painkillers become dangerous: what everyone needs to know about OxyCotin and other prescription pain medications*. New York: Hazelden.

Piper, M.C., Kunos, V.I., Willis, D.M., Mazer, B.L., Ramsay, M. & Silver, K.M. (1986). Early physical therapy effects on the high-risk infant: a randomized controlled trial. *Pediatrics*, 78(2), 216-224.

Radomski, M.V., & Trombly, C.A., (2008). *Occupational therapy for physical dysfunction*. New York: Lippencott, Williams & Wilkins.

Scadding, J.W. (1992). Neuropathic pain. *ACNR*, 3(2), 8-14.

Seidenberg, A.B. & An, Y.H. (2003). Is there an inhibitory effect of COX-2 inhibitors on bone

healing? *Pharmacological Research*, 50, 151-156.

Sinclair, S., Hogg-Johnson, S., Mondloch, M.V., & Shields, S.A. (1997). The effectiveness of an early active intervention program for workers with soft tissue injuries: the early claimant cohort study. *Spine*, 22(24), 2919-2931.

Smith, H.S., Audette, J, & Royal, M.A. (2002). Botulinum toxin in pain management of soft tissue syndromes. *Clinical Journal of Pain*, 18(6), S147-S154.

Stanish, W.D., (1984). Overuse injuries in athletes: a perspective. *Medicine & Science in Sports & Exercise*, 16(1), 1-7.

Stevens, D.L, Bisno, A.L., Chambers, H.F., Everette, E.D., Dellinger, P, Goldstein, E.J.C., et al. (2005). Practice guidelines for the diagnosis and management of skin and soft-tissue infections. *Clinical Infectious Diseases*, 41, 1373-1406.

Taylor, N.F., Dodd., K.J., & Damiano, D.L., (2006). Progressive resistance exercise in physical therapy: a summary of systematic review. *Physical Therapy*, 85(11), 1208-1223.

Von Roenn, J.H., Cleeland, C.S., Gonin, R., Hatfield, A.K., & Pandya, K.J. (1993). Physician attitudes and practice in cancer pain management: A survey from the Eastern Cooperative Oncology Group. *Annals of Internal Medicine*, 119(2), 121-126.

Wallace, M.S. & Staats, P. *Pain Medicine and Management: Just the facts*. New York: McGraw-Hill Professional.

Wallis, B.J., Lord, S.M., Barnsley, L, & Bogduk, N. (1996). Pain and psychological symptoms of Australian patients with whiplash. *Spine*, 21(7), 804-810.

Ward, S.E., Goldberg, N., Miller-McCauley, V., Mueller, C., Nolan, A., Pawlik-Plank, D., et.al (1993). Patient-related barriers to management of cancer pain. *Pain*, 52(3), 319-324.

Warfield, C.A., & Kahn, C.H. (1995). Acute pain management: Program in U.S. hospitals and experiences and attitudes among U.S. adults. *Anesthesiology*, 83(5), 1090-1094. Warfield, C., & Bajwa, Z. (2004). *Principles and practice of pain medicines*. New York: McGraw Hill Professional.

Weber, M.D., Servedio, F.J., & Woodall, W.R., (1994). The effects of three modalities on delayed onset muscle soreness. *Journal of Orthopedic and Sports Physical Therapy*, 20(5), 236-242.

Wolff, B.B. (2005). A brief history of pain from a personal perspective. In M.V. Boswell & B.E. Cole (Eds.) *Weiner's Pain Management: A practical guide for clinicians*. New York: Informa Health Care.

Yeung, E.W., & Yeung, S.S., (2001). A systematic review of interventions to prevent lower limb soft tissue running injuries. *British Journal of Sports Medicine*, 35(10), 383-389.

www.ingramcontent.com/pod-product-compliance
Lightning Source LLC
Chambersburg PA
CBHW070948200526
45161CB00001BA/32